Epilepsy in Young People

Epilepsy in Young People

Portsmouth Symposium,
June, 1986

Edited by

EUAN ROSS
Charing Cross Hospital, London, UK

DAVID CHADWICK
Walton Hospital, Liverpool, UK
and
ROBERT CRAWFORD
Ciba-Geigy Pharmaceuticals, Horsham, UK

A Wiley Medical Publication

JOHN WILEY & SONS
Chichester · New York · Brisbane · Toronto · Singapore

Library of Congress Cataloging-in-Publication Data:

Epilepsy in young people.

(A Wiley medical publication)
Cataloging in publication.
Includes index.
1. Epilepsy in youth—Congresses. 2. Epilepsy in
children—Congresses. I. Ross, Euan M.
II. Crawford, Robert, 1956- . III. Chadwick, David.
[DNLM: 1. Epilepsy—in adolescence—congresses.
WL 385 E64128 1986]
RJ496.E6E652 1987 618.92′853 86-32590
ISBN 0 471 91469 X

British Library Cataloguing in Publication Data:

Epilepsy in young people: symposium held at
the Holiday Inn, Portsmouth, June 1986.
1. Epilepsy in children
I. Ross, Euan II. Chadwick, David
III. Crawford, Robert
616.8′53 RJ496.E6

ISBN 0 471 91469 X

Printed and bound in Great Britain.

Contents

Chairmen and Contributors

Christopher B. T. Adams, *Radcliffe Infirmary, Oxford*

Martin J. Brodie, *Western Infirmary, Glasgow*

Julie Bullen, *King's College Hospital, London*

David W. Chadwick, *Walton Hospital, Liverpool*

Pamela M. Crawford, *North Manchester General Hospital*

Graham F. A. Harding, *Aston University, Birmingham*

Peter M. Jeavons, *Aston University, Birmingham*

Zarrina Kurtz, *Institute of Child Health, London*

Janet Lindsay, *Park Hospital for Children, Oxford*

Ian McKinlay, *Booth Hall Hospital, Manchester*

Jolyon R. Oxley, *National Society for Epilepsy, Chalfont Centre for Epilepsy, Buckinghamshire*

Theresa E. Powell, *Aston University, Birmingham*

Peter J. Rogan, *St Michael's Primary School, Knowsley, Merseyside*

Euan M. Ross, *Charing Cross Hospital, London*

Simon D. Shorvon, *National Hospitals for Nervous Diseases, London*

John Stephenson, *Royal Hospital for Sick Children, Glasgow*

Gregory Stores, *Park Hospital for Children, Oxford*

Leonard Thornton, *Royal Manchester Children's Hospital*

Pat Tookey, *Institute of Child Health, London*

Michael R. Trimble, *National Hospitals for Nervous Diseases, London*

Sheila J. Wallace, *University Hospital of Wales, Cardiff*

Arnold J. Wilkins, *MRC Applied Psychology Unit, Cambridge*

Preface

This book brings together papers from a conference held in Portsmouth in the summer of 1986. It is the second such report that Ciba-Geigy have sponsored, following *Paediatric Perspectives on Epilepsy*, published in 1985. This time our perspectives shifted to cover the older child, school leavers and young adults.

Do read the pickled version of the lively discussion between the papers: together with more concise style and speedier publication, they mark the real difference between this type of book and a conventional textbook that takes several years' gestation. It was neither possible nor desirable to avoid some overlap between papers because epilepsy cannot be subdivided into neat self-contained series of problems. If our writers have reflected the current mixture of hope and pessimism that pervades the understanding of epilepsy in young people, we will be satisfied. Like manufacturers of chocolates we have included contents with varying degrees of hardness though none are soft-centred. On publication, this book should provide up-to-date information for all concerned with the care of young people with epilepsy. We hope that it will keep well, and with age be useful as a record of informed thought on the subject that was current in 1986.

EUAN ROSS
DAVID CHADWICK
ROBERT CRAWFORD

Acknowledgements

Dr George Birdwood undertook the detailed preparation of this book, and the volume editors and publisher would like to express their gratitude for his enthusiastic hard work.

Section I: Social implications

Epilepsy in Young People
Edited by E. Ross, D. Chadwick and R. Crawford

1

Epilepsy care: the problem from child to adult

IAN McKINLAY
Booth Hall Hospital, Manchester

SUMMARY

Epilepsy is the commonest neurological problem in adolescence, usually with serious consequences for this most critical period of development. In terms of incidence, the average GP will have between six and eight severely mentally handicapped patients in the practice, of whom between one and three will be children or adolescents with a seizure disorder. Evaluating the effectiveness of care is essential. School grade in relation to age has been found to be a better predictor of overall family, social and academic function in the epileptic patient than neurological impairment.

Liability to seizures modifies leisure choices, social status and sexual partners. Families have a crucial responsibility to ensure that their offspring can make their way in the world. Therefore both adolescents and parents need information about epilepsy and its consequences, advice on treatment and details of prognosis. Any potential abilities should be actively developed to give every child with epilepsy hope for the future.

INTRODUCTION

Adolescents with epilepsy face special problems as well as the usual opportunities that all young people go through as they grow up. They are developing an integrated view of themselves, becoming independent through social and sexual development, leaving home and school, and competing for jobs or places in further education. Many want to take part in sport and other recreation, to travel and to drive. All become eligible to drink alcohol in public places, to vote, and to marry and raise a family. It is an exciting but insecure time. Freedom is constrained by responsibility. For those with a neurological impairment the meaning of chronicity with its future implications dawns first during adolescence (Graham, 1985).

PREVALENCE

Epilepsy is the most common neurological problem in adolescence. Cooper (1965) reported 4.7 new and 3.4 old cases per 1000 at age 15 (total prevalence 8.2/1000). Castle and Fishman (1973) found that 63% of adolescents with neurological problems (and 9.9% of all adolescents seen in their clinic) attended because of epilepsy. Garell (1965) found epilepsy to be among the top five conditions in adolescent clinic attenders in Canada and the USA.

PROGNOSIS

Some seizure disorders cease or improve during puberty, some persist, some become worse and some change. New seizure disorders emerge (Juul-Jensen and Foldspang, 1983; Cavazutti, 1980). Primary generalized epilepsy of petit mal type usually ceases or improves. In a small number, primary generalized grand mal seizures emerge. Benign focal epilepsy remits during puberty and does not seem to relapse later (Blom and Heijbel, 1982). Photic hypersensitivity usually commences in early puberty and continues for about ten years (Jeavons and Harding, 1975). Primary generalized epilepsy with grand mal on waking (at any time of day) or when relaxing in the evening usually begins during puberty. It is usually idiopathic, though a genetic predisposition is frequent, and there is a link with photosensitivity (Wolf, 1985a). Myoclonic epilepsy of adolescence (Aicardi and Chevrie, 1971) consists of bilateral jerking, often repetitive, of the shoulders and arms usually shortly after waking. It is more common in girls, and attacks may occur during menstruation. This may be associated with juvenile absence epilepsy (Wolf, 1985b), and sporadic generalized seizures which respond well to treatment. Benign partial seizures of adolescence (Loiseau and Louiset, 1985) have an onset at 10–20 years (peak 13–14 years). They may be simple or complex with motor and/or sensory symptoms, frequently with secondary generalization, occurring singly or in clusters and predominantly in otherwise healthy boys without a family history. Partial seizures secondary to demonstrable lesions may declare themselves, sometimes leading to surgical treatment and the problems of rehabilitation it entails (Meyer *et al.*, 1986). Other seizure disorders become worse, such as Lennox-Gastaut syndrome, and those associated with autism or severe mental handicap. In a personal survey of 154 mentally handicapped schoolchildren in Salford (Fig. 1), 53 were found to suffer from epilepsy (34.4%) with a slightly higher proportion in boys (36.2% vs 31.7% for girls). The proportion of those with epilepsy under ten years of age was 26.7%, but for those over ten the proportion was 39.4%.

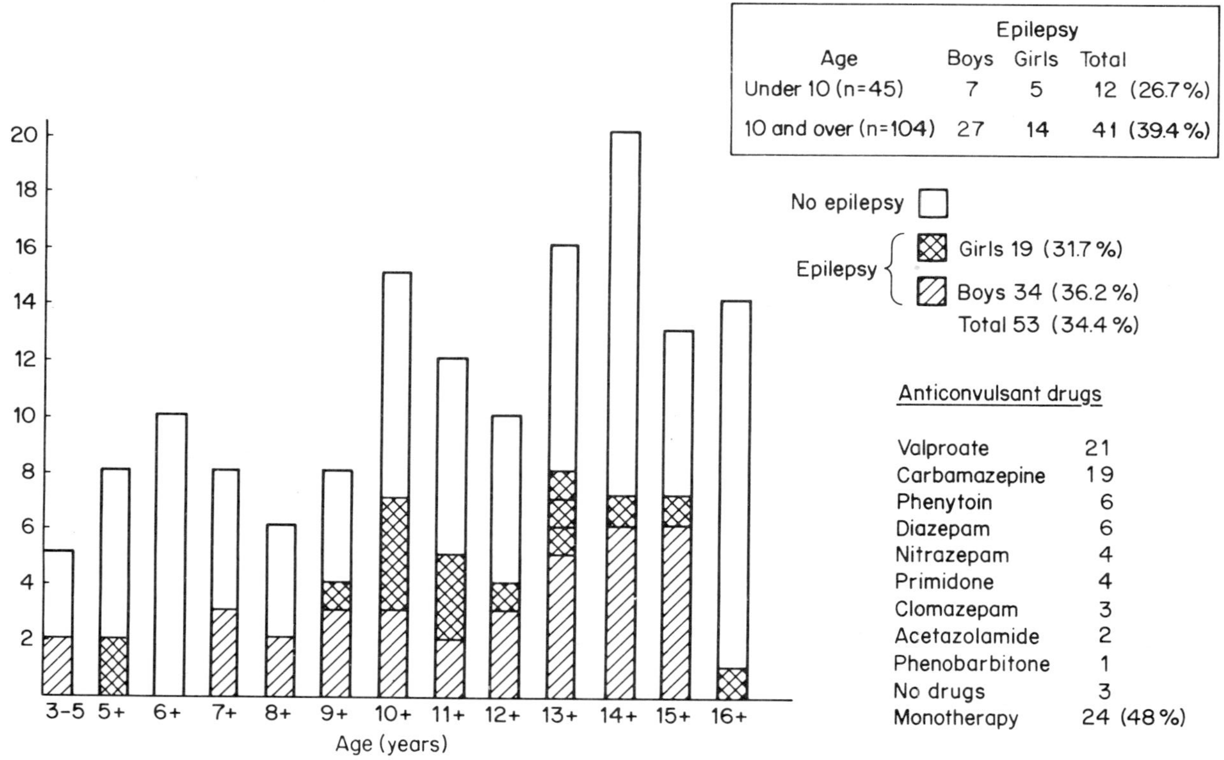

Fig. 1 Prevalence of epilepsy by age among 154 educationally subnormal schoolchildren in Salford, 1983

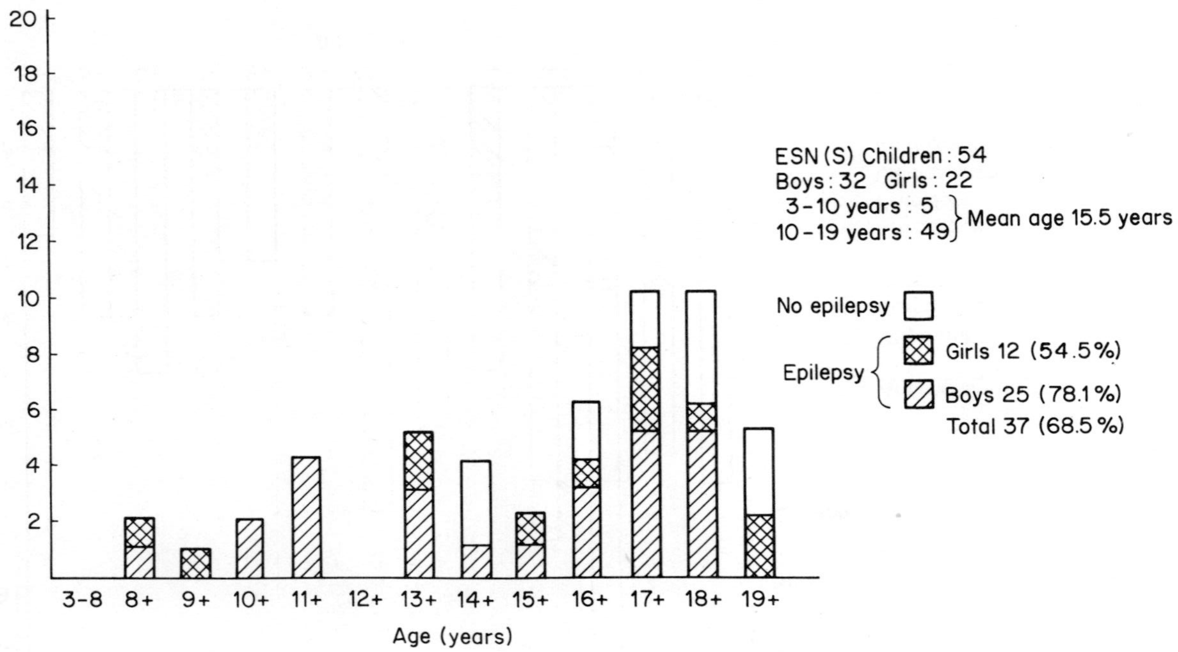

Fig. 2 Prevalence of epilepsy by age among 54 educationally subnormal schoolchildren attending Queen Mary's Hospital, Carshalton, 1984

In a parallel study of mentally handicapped children in institutional care at Queen Mary's Hospital, Carshalton, the proportion with epilepsy was 68.5% (Fig. 2), suggesting that epilepsy is a factor which limits the ability of families to cope with mentally handicapped members. This has powerful implications for 'care in the community' if these institutions are to be abolished in the near future. A general practitioner with an average size list will have between six and eight severely mentally handicapped patients of whom five are likely to be adults and two or three will have a seizure disorder. It is fashionable to assert that mentally handicapped people have as much right to general services as anyone else. Evaluating the effectiveness of care will be necessary. Inarticulate patients being treated by inexperienced doctors may be at risk of prolonged exposure to drugs which prove ineffective and produce unnecessary side-effects.

TREATMENT

It is to be expected that adolescents will become more independent of hospital clinics and more able to ask their general practitioners for help if need be. However, a single outpatient visit may not be enough, if the seizure disorder is of recent onset, has increased in severity, or affects a patient with impaired communication. It may be as much as some neurologists or physicians can offer though. There is a case for providing an adult neurological rehabilitation service in each health district to offer continuity of advice for the general practitioner as well as the patient. For handicapped adults in Britain, systematic health care monitoring in training centres or other facilities should be carried out by a senior clinical medical officer from the community health service. Liaison with general practitioners is essential, and specialist services can be involved as required. In other authorities a specialist in mental handicap or psychiatry or interested general practitioners may provide the service. This lack of a planned service is a cause of concern for families of adolescents who have been accustomed to paediatric review.

In a study of 445 patients with epilepsy over the age of 15, Ryan *et al.* (1980) found there was no universal feeling of being stigmatized. Their perception of stigma depended less directly on the severity of seizures than on educational attainments, limitations imposed by their disorder and the realization that there might be discrimination when seeking employment. Ziegler (1981) discussed the way in which epilepsy disrupts the patient's and parent's sense of control and competence, making autonomy more difficult. Hoare (1984) found that excessive dependence and psychiatric disorder were more common in children who developed epilepsy than in those with diabetes. Kellerman *et al.* (1980) and Zeltzer *et al.* (1980) studied 168 adolescents with diabetes, cystic fibrosis, cancer, cardiac, renal or rheumatological diseases, compared with 349 controls, and found no difference in anxiety, self-esteem or reaction to illness between groups or within the categories in the afflicted groups. However, Hodgman *et al.* (1979)

found low self-esteem and poor expectation for the future in adolescents with epilepsy, particularly in those (irrespective of IQ or school performance) without associated (stigmatizing) neurological defects. School grade in relation to age was a better predictor of overall family social and academic function than neurological impairment. The difference between the consequences of general physical and neurological disorders has been apparent for centuries (e.g. Hill, 1981). Social attitudes contribute to this. In a Nigerian study (Awaritefe *et al.*, 1985) the literate general public had a much more negative attitude to people with epilepsy than to 'cured' psychotic people. Taylor (1971) suggests that temporal lobe abnormalities may impede the development of personal identity.

CONSTRAINTS DUE TO EPILEPSY

There are many potential constraints for adolescents with epilepsy. Career opportunities and driving licences are restricted by regulation. Drug effects may modify dexterity and could affect exam results. 'Having seizures' modifies leisure choices, and social and sexual partners. Excessive alcohol intake provokes seizures, though moderate drinking does not (Hillbom, 1980; Hoppener *et al.*, 1983). Exercise seems to have a protective effect, but seizures may occur afterwards (Kuyer, 1977). Going without sleep and irregular hours are part of teenage culture but may encourage seizures. Some anticonvulsants interact with contraceptives and there are small teratogenic risks. Women with epilepsy have higher rates of both pregnancy complications and low-birth-weight babies (Yerby *et al.*, 1985). There is a small excess risk in most cases, but adolescents of normal intelligence with tuberous sclerosis are bound to have a great deal of anxiety despite counselling. Caring for a baby is more difficult if a parent is liable to have seizures. Most of these problems can be overcome but they need to be remembered. Rehabilitation programmes have been shown to improve job prospects (Fraser *et al.*, 1983). Advice on availability of drugs and immigration laws will be needed by some who travel abroad.

ADVICE TO THE FAMILY

Families have a crucial responsibility in helping their young people to make their way. A worthwhile occupation, a sense of being cared for, a conviction that others have faith in one's future, leisure activities to look forward to and knowing that someone will listen all facilitate the development of self-confidence. To foster such evolution for a young person who is sometimes argumentative, irresponsible, boisterous, sullen, demanding, touchy and apparently ungrateful demands a good deal of good humour from parents who, themselves, may have problems in mid-life. Parents enjoy their children's success and the sharing of some of their activities, but must also allow them some privacy and avoid excessive control.

Both adolescents and their parents need information about epilepsy and its consequences, and advice on treatment and prognosis to help them negotiate their own way. They may have difficulty in knowing the questions to ask as the experience is novel. The tendency has been for doctors to talk *about* adolescents to their parents rather than to engage the young people themselves in making decisions. How little many patients understand about epilepsy or its treatment after years of clinic attendance! Doctors conducting busy clinics will be familiar with the apparent apathy of their adolescent patients. Doctors and patients know such clinics are first-aid stations. How can this be overcome?

First, a doctor or an informed member of the team such as a nurse, social worker or psychologist can make time to talk to the patient. It can be revealing to ask 'Do you understand what epilepsy is and what your treatment is for?' Choices can be offered so far as treatment is concerned. Schools can become involved (Gadow, 1982; Freeman *et al.*, 1984). Self-help groups can be promoted. No doubt one of the benefits for children attending special centres is the opportunity to meet similarly affected peers. In our own department it is interesting to observe how readily adolescent patients will answer a questionnaire about epilepsy and its treatment. Willingness to write references on behalf of a patient indicates whose side the doctor is on. Perhaps the greatest area of neglect is management of the transition to adult services, which have much less capacity to take a continuing personal interest in 'routine cases'. One way to proceed would be to have clinics for adolescents in each district involving both child and adult specialists. Another is to arrange phased transfer where the patient will visit the adult clinic then return to the paediatric clinic for discussion. We offer a home visit by our social worker prior to discharge to tie up any 'loose ends', though social work departments tend to accord low priority to such work. When the transfer is made it is courteous to send a comprehensive summary to the adult specialist.

OUTLOOK

Although children with epilepsy should be reviewed regularly, impending discharge is a special stimulus for review of the diagnosis and treatment. Not every 'known epileptic' has epilepsy. Some drug treatments are ineffective or unnecessary (Thurston *et al.*, 1982; Todt, 1984) for particular patients. Selective surgery has a definite place well before school-leaving age. Psychiatric health is an essential component of management and physicians may need to consider greater involvement of adolescent psychiatry in their epilepsy services to prevent later crises. Emotional well-being facilitates seizure control, and putting to full use the abilities of adolescents can induce in them an optimistic outlook for the future.

REFERENCES

AICARDI, J. and CHEVRIE, J. J. (1971) Myoclonic epilepsies of childhood. *Neuropaediatrie*, **3**, 177–190.

AWARITEFE, A., LONGE, A. C. and AWARITEFE, M. (1985) Epilepsy and psychosis: A comparison of societal attitudes. *Epilepsia*, **26**, 1–9.

BLOM, S. and HEIJBEL, J. (1982) Benign epilepsy of children with centrotemporal EEG foci: a follow-up study in adulthood of patients initially studied as children. *Epilepsia*, **23**, 629–632.

CASTLE, G. F. and FISHMAN, L. S. (1973) Seizures in adolescent medicine. *Pediatr. Clin. North Am.*, **20**, 819–835.

CAVAZUTTI, G. B. (1980) Epidemiology of different types of epilepsy in school age children of Modena, Italy. *Epilepsia*, **21**, 57–62.

COOPER, J. E. (1965) Epilepsy in a longitudinal survey of 5000 children. *Br. Med. J.*, **1**, 1020–1022.

FRASER, R. T., CLEMMONS, D., TREJO, W. and TEMKIN, N. R. (1983) Program evaluation in epilepsy rehabilitation. *Epilepsia*, **24**, 734–746.

FREEMAN, J. M., JACOBS, H., VINING, E. and RABIN, C. E. (1984) Epilepsy and inner city schools: A school-based program that makes a difference. *Epilepsia*, **21**, 261–271.

GADOW, K. D. (1982) School involvement in the treatment of seizure disorders. *Epilepsia*, **23**, 215–224.

GARELL, D. C. (1965) A Survey of adolescent medicine in the US and Canada. *Am. J. Dis. Child.*, **109**, 314–317.

GRAHAM, P. (1985) Handling stress in the handicapped adolescent. *Dev. Med. Child Neurol.*, **27**, 389–391.

HILL, D. D. (1982) Historical Review. In: *Epilepsy and Psychiatry*, E. H. Reynolds and M. R. Trimble (Eds), Churchill Livingstone, Edinburgh, pp. 1–11.

HILLBOM, M. E. (1980) Occurrence of cerebral seizures provoked by alcohol abuse. *Epilepsia*, **21**, 459–466.

HOARE, P. (1984) Does illness foster dependency? A study of epileptic and diabetic children. *Dev. Med. Child Neurol.*, **26**, 20–24.

HODGMAN, C. H., MCANARNEY, E. R., MYERS, G. J., IKER, H., MCKINNEY, R., PARMELEC, D., SCHUSTER, B. and TUTIHASI, M. (1979) Emotional complications of adolescent grand mal epilepsy. *J. Pediatr.*, **95**, 309–312.

HOPPENER, R. J., KUYER, A. and VAN DER LUGT, P. J. M. (1983) Epilepsy and alcohol: the influence of social alcohol intake on seizures and treatment in epilepsy. *Epilepsia*, **24**, 459–471.

JEAVONS, P. and HARDING, G. F. A. (1975) Photosensitive epilepsy: Prognosis. *Clinics in Developmental Medicine*, vol. 56, Spastics International Medical Publications, Heinemann Medical, London, pp. 103–104.

JUUL-JENSEN, P. and FOLDSPANG, A. (1983) Natural history of epileptic seizures. *Epilepsia*, **24**, 297–312.

KELLERMAN, J., ZELTZER, L., ELLENBERG, L., DASH, J. and RIGLER, D. (1980) Psychological effects of illness in adolescence. I. Anxiety, self-esteem and perception of control. *J. Pediatr.*, **97**, 126–131.

KUYER, A. (1977) *Epilepsy and Exercise*, S.R.A.E. Meer en Bosche, Heemstede.

LOISEAU, P. and LOUISET, P. (1985) Benign partial seizures of adolescence. In: *Epileptic Syndromes in Infancy, Childhood and Adolescence*, J. Roger *et al.* (Eds), John Libbey Eurotext, London, pp. 274–277.

MEYER, F. B., MARSH, R., LAWS, E. R. and SHARBROUGH, F. W. (1986) Temporal lobectomy in children with epilepsy. *J. Neurosurg.*, **64**, 371–376.

RYAN, R., KEMPNER, K. and EMLEN, A. C. (1980) The stigma of epilepsy as a self concept. *Epilepsia*, **21**, 433–444.

TAYLOR, D. C. (1971) Psychiatry and sociology in the understanding of epilepsy. In: *Psychiatric Aspects of Medical Practice*, M. G. Gelder and B. M. Mandelbrote (Eds), Staples, London, pp. 161–186.

THURSTON, J. H., THURSTON, D. L., HIXON, B. B. and KELLER, A. J. (1982) Prognosis in childhood epilepsy: Additional follow-up of 148 children 15 to 23 years after withdrawal of anticonvulsant therapy. *N. Engl. J. Med.*, **306**, 831–836.

TODT, H. (1984) The late prognosis of epilepsy in childhood: Results of a prospective follow-up study. *Epilepsia*, **25**, 137–144.

WOLF, P. (1985a) Epilepsy with grand mal on awakening. In: *Epileptic Syndromes in Infancy, Childhood and Adolescence*, J. Roger *et al.* (Eds), John Libbey Eurotext, London, pp. 259–270.

WOLF, P. (1985b) Juvenile absence epilepsy. In: *Epileptic Syndromes in Infancy, Childhood and Adolescence*, J. Roger *et al.* (Eds), John Libbey Eurotext, London, pp. 242–246.

YERBY, M., KOEPSELL, T. and DALING, J. (1985) Pregnancy complications and outcomes in a cohort of women with epilepsy. *Epilepsia*, **26**, 631–635.

ZELTZER, L., KELLERMAN, J., ELLENBERG, L., DASH, J. and RIGLER, D. (1980) Psychological effects of illness in adolescence. II. Impact of illness in adolescents—crucial issues and coping styles. *J. Pediatr.*, **97**, 132–138.

ZIEGLER, R. G. (1981) Impairments of control and competence in epileptic children and their families. *Epilepsia*, **22**, 339–346.

DISCUSSION

Dr J. Stephenson (Glasgow): Do you think the word epilepsy should be used for the benign focal seizures of adolescents? These seizures may be single or clustered within a week or so, but this differs from epilepsy as usually defined and does not have the same implications.

McKinlay: The episodes are probably brain-initiated phenomena and need not be excluded from the whole concept of epilepsy just because they are mild with EEG findings that are often fairly slight. I would accept that single seizures or a cluster of seizures within a week or so need not be considered as epilepsy.

Dr M. Noronha (Manchester): One of the big problems that we face is the transition from childhood epilepsy to adult life. How can we pass them on to suitable agencies for their ongoing care?

McKinlay: This is probably the biggest management issue in child health services at present. For young people with associated neurological impairments, mental handicap and cerebral palsy, the main needs are for a rehabilitation service and for a review of day care facilities. Adult neurology services are very willing to give one-off opinions but not equipped for long-term follow-up. At the same time, many general practitioners do not feel confident to manage these disorders year-by-year, although some will be. There is definitely a case for developing a neurological rehabilitation service to take an active interest in such patients throughout their adult lives. The rheumatology type of rehabilitation is not really suitable, and I would like to see a substantial development of facilities for adult neurological rehabilitation. In some health districts, individual psychiatrists, including mental handicap psychiatrists, may be able and willing to treat people with epilepsy; in others, an interested group of general practitioners provide such services, but provision needs to be planned and generally available.

Noronha: After years of looking after mentally-handicapped children with epilepsy, we too often see them come unstuck immediately they're passed on to adult services.

McKinlay: That's true, partly because the seizure disorders are often changing around the time we pass them on. On the whole, the mental handicap specialists concentrate more on psychiatry than on epilepsy, although some individuals are interested in epilepsy.

Dr E. M. Ross (London), Chairman: Can anybody here give an example of good practice or innovative ideas that may help to overcome these problems?

Dr D. R. Knight (Northampton): I'm a psychiatrist and also responsible for an EEG department. For the last ten years I have been running a combined paediatric epilepsy clinic with a paediatrician. When the patients reach 16, they become mine, as I run the adolescent clinic and also look after handicap. This is one way of keeping continuity.

Ross: We tried to do this at Central Middlesex Hospital by running a children's epilepsy clinic in the EEG department with the adult neurologist. We were able to show the EEG to children when it was being done, the technicians got to know the children too, and the child psychiatry department was next door.

Dr J. Corbett (London): One of the important things to come out of our research following up children into adult life is the need to know what happened to them in childhood. With all due respect to the paediatricians present, the records don't always tell you what drugs the children have had and what their seizure frequency was from month to month. Alan Richens has devised a technique for summarizing seizures, and the annual summary charts are now available. These are most helpful when you meet somebody for the first time in adolescence and it is necessary to reassess educational and medical needs for the future.

Epilepsy in Young People
Edited by E. Ross, D. Chadwick and R. Crawford

2

The epidemiology of epilepsy in childhood

ZARRINA KURTZ* (speaker), PAT TOOKEY* and EUAN ROSS†
Institute of Child Health, London, and †Charing Cross Hospital, London

SUMMARY

Epidemiological studies provide information on the prevalence, incidence, causal factors and natural history of epilepsy in childhood, but rates vary depending on the way in which epilepsy is defined, on the completeness of case-finding and on the populations studied. Information is presented and discussed from cross-sectional and longitudinal studies on clinic, general practice, school, local and national populations.

In a nationally representative cohort of children born in one week in 1958 in England, Scotland and Wales 4.1 per 1000 had a history of epilepsy up to the age of 11, according to defined criteria. Preliminary data are given from follow-up of the cohort at the ages of 16 and 23, on the natural history of epilepsy in these children and on the occurrence of new cases. Aspects including the proportion of children who become free of fits, the proportion for whom the cause of epilepsy is known, and the proportion who have additional handicaps are discussed in the light of other studies.

INTRODUCTION

Epidemiology has the potential to answer some of the questions we most want to ask about epilepsy in childhood. These include how common it is, and whether it is becoming more so; whether the incidence and prevalence vary at different ages, and in different localities; what are the likely, and the rare, causes; whether certain children are more likely to develop epilepsy, and how certainly we can make predictions; what types of epilepsy we may expect in childhood, their natural histories, and rates of secondary handicap—educational, behavioural and socioeconomic—as well as the identification of risk factors. These are questions that clinicians cannot answer from their own experience alone, and even pooled experience is likely to combine selection bias in cases and catchment populations. Answers are needed to advise parents on prognosis, to improve efforts at prevention, and to plan services both for children with epilepsy and for their families.

Such questions cost a great deal of time, money and effort to answer. They are only worth studying if there is a reasonable chance that the findings can be correctly interpreted. This will depend on an exact definition of what is taken as a 'case' of epilepsy, on finding all cases, and on a detailed description of the population from which they are drawn. Otherwise we merely make lists that may mislead.

PREVALENCE

Case definition

It is well recognized that the rate of epilepsy found in child population studies varies according to the definition used. In a review of over 30 reports, Rose *et al.* (1973) found rates varying from 150 per 1000 children in the tropical island of Guam to 1.5 per 1000 in Japanese schoolchildren. Even in European and North American populations, the rates vary between 3.2 and 7.2 per 1000 (Ross and Peckham, 1983). These may reflect true differences in the rates of disease, but how can we be sure when different criteria for inclusion of children with epilepsy are used in different studies? On the whole, higher rates are found where relatively relaxed criteria for epilepsy are accepted. In Cooper's study (1965) of 11-year-olds in England, Scotland and Wales, there was a prevalence of 7.1 per 1000 when epilepsy was defined as 'a fit or convulsion during the previous year reported by mothers of children over the age of two years and confirmed as epilepsy at examination by school medical officers'. In the Isle of Wight, Rutter *et al.* (1970) found a rate of 7.2 per 1000 when 'a child must have had a definite fit since he started school, and during the previous 12 months there must have been either a fit or the child must have taken regular anticonvulsants'. In Camberwell (Kangesu, 1984) with a rate of 3.4 per 1000, children were identified from the Community Child Health Services Handicap Register and their diagnosis confirmed from medical records.

These different study definitions reflect the difficulties experienced by clinicians working with children who have epilepsy in deciding whether a child's problems really have an epileptic basis. Decisions rest on clinical judgements, and eyewitness accounts of seizures are needed. There are no characteristic physical signs, and diagnostic aids such as the EEG are not always helpful. Because no two studies have adopted the same definitions, there remains a barrier in interpreting the findings for the rates of epilepsy associated with age groups, geographical locations, and the year of research in different studies.

Case finding

The way in which patients are recruited also influences the rates. Prevalence rates for children with epilepsy have been obtained from surveys of those attending hospital, of general practice populations and of schools. Even in developed countries, where it is generally assumed that most children with epilepsy will be investigated or treated at hospital at some time in their lives, there is conflicting evidence about the proportion who attend. Crombie *et al.* (1960) reported that 75% of patients with epilepsy saw only general practitioners; in contrast the Carlisle population study (Brewis *et al.*, 1966), carried out in a similar period, found that 78% had seen specialists. Children attending a particular hospital or clinic may show special characteristics and will almost certainly present more serious and intractable problems than would be encountered if the whole community were studied. Even comprehensive studies, such as those from the Mayo Clinic in the USA (Hauser and Kurland, 1975), suffer from this problem.

General practice studies tend to exclude the most seriously affected children who may be hidden in long-term residential institutions. Neither hospital nor general practice based studies have access to those who do not seek treatment. General practice studies, carried out separately by Pond *et al.* (1960) and Crombie *et al.* (1960), found differing rates in prevalence between practices that probably reflected variations in notification. More recently, Goodridge and Shorvon (1983) reviewed epilepsy in patients in general practice in Tonbridge. They found 20 cases of epilepsy among 1612 children and adolescents under the age of 20 years in a practice population of 6000, giving a prevalence of 12.4 per 1000. Among patients of all ages with epilepsy 56% said their fits had started before the age of ten years. Recently, Goodridge has been instrumental in setting up a national general practice study which will give greater insight into the early stages of epilepsy and the ways in which it is managed by general practitioners.

There have been a number of studies based on school populations (Holdsworth and Whitmore, 1974; Kangesu *et al.*, 1984). It cannot be assumed that school-based studies will identify all children with epilepsy. Until the 1970 Education Act came into force, some children with epilepsy were not attending school (Kurtz, 1983). Nowadays the majority of children with epilepsy attend ordinary schools. In Kangesu's study of schoolchildren aged 5–15 years in southeast London, 50 of the 92 children with epilepsy in a population of 27 000 were attending ordinary school. It has been estimated that education authorities may know of as few as half the children with epilepsy in school (DHSS, 1969). In addition, children may remain on education authority records as having epilepsy for variable lengths of time after they have stopped having seizures. Those in special schools may be placed outside their local area. A small and shrinking proportion of children with multiple handicaps attend residential special schools for epilepsy, but others attend day and residential special schools for the physically handicapped, educationally subnormal, or maladjusted. In these situations, it is often not recorded that they have epilepsy: for example, surveys of special schools have reported seizures in 25% of cerebral palsied children and in 5–8% of visually handicapped children (Ingram and Fine, quoted by Gulliford, 1971).

It is difficult to tell whether the prevalence of epilepsy is changing over time because of the different definitions and the different populations studied. However, the 1958 and 1970 British birth cohorts used similar definitions of epilepsy and do not show any change in the prevalence of epilepsy in childhood.

New techniques for studying brain activity can show epileptic changes without evidence of fits. If these techniques become more widespread the proportion of children revealed as having some kind of epilepsy is likely to increase.

NATURAL HISTORY

It is not possible to obtain information on the natural history of epilepsy or fits in childhood from cross-sectional studies. Longitudinal studies, which follow children over a period of time, are required. Apart from the Mayo Clinic series in the US there are few longitudinal studies of epilepsy from childhood through to adolescence, let alone to adult life. These have mostly been clinic-based follow-ups such as that by Kiorboe in Denmark (1961). In Britain, Harrison and Taylor (1976) reported a 25-year review of 207 children with fits of all kinds, based on clinic attendances in the Oxford region. These series may give different prognoses from studies based on geographically defined populations.

The United Kingdom is unique in having carried out three longitudinal studies of child development based on one-week cohorts of children born in 1946, 1958 and 1970. In each of these years, all infants born in a selected spring week were studied in detail from birth. All three studies have investigated children with epilepsy as special substudies and have provided much useful information about this condition in unselected children. The National Childhood Encephalopathy Study (Miller *et al.*, 1981) was set up to study serious neurological disorder in children aged 2–35 months in relation to immunization; this has also gathered a great deal of data on the antecedents of epilepsy in a national population. The longitudinal studies of children's epilepsies have been discussed by Verity and Ross (1985).

The National Child Development Study epilepsy follow-up

The natural history of epilepsy in children is discussed here in relation to the National Child Development Study (NCDS) which followed all 17 733 children born in the week 3–9 March in England, Scotland and Wales in 1958. In the week of their birth their antenatal and perinatal histories were recorded. Subsequently, the survivors were traced at the ages of 7, 11 and 16 and their parents were visited by health visitors who obtained details of their family, social and medical background. At school, they were medically examined and their school performance assessed. At the age of 23, members of the cohort were again traced to their homes and interviews were carried out to obtain family, social, medical and employment details. Among data gathered on each occasion were facts about the occurrence of seizures. When the children were 13 years old a substudy of those with possible epilepsy was undertaken, based on data collected at birth and from the 7- and 11-year-old follow-up (Ross *et al.*, 1980).

Of the 15 496 of the original children who were traced and alive at age 11, a history of at least one seizure or episode of altered consciousness was obtained in 1043; their records were carefully scrutinized. Those who satisfied the study definition of epilepsy as 'recurrent paroxysmal disturbance of consciousness, sensation or movement, primarily cerebral in origin, unassociated with acute febrile episodes' were divided into three groups: those who had febrile convulsions only (346), those who had fits before the age of five only and those who had at least one non-febrile fit after five. The children in this latter subgroup were regarded as the most likely to have epilepsy and they were studied intensively using information obtained from questionnaires completed by family doctors and hospital and community specialists.

At the age of 11, there was a prevalence of epilepsy of 4.1 per 1000 in this national population which comprised 64 children. A further 39 had epilepsy as reported by a doctor, but they did not meet the study definition criteria. Twenty of the children in the cohort who had had febrile convulsions went on to have a non-febrile seizure, a rate of 5%; the rate was only 0.5% in those children with febrile convulsions managed entirely at home but increased to 15% among children admitted to hospital. Ross and Peckham (1983) have discussed these findings and those from other studies with regard to the prevalence and prognosis of febrile convulsions and the relationship with epilepsy in childhood.

We have now scrutinized all the information gathered at the 23-year follow-up. Those with any evidence of epilepsy either reported then for the first time or revealed in the earlier phases of the study are being investigated further. With permission from the survey respondents we are contacting the doctors involved in order to validate the diagnosis. We will interview all those with epilepsy to obtain information about aspects of their health, medical supervision, employment and quality of life. We hope to obtain incidence rates for new cases arising at different ages, to build up a picture of the effects of epilepsy in childhood on adult life, and to shed light on why and when epilepsy remits and why it does not.

Preliminary analysis of this study shows that at the 16-year-old follow-up 1636 (14% of the cohort) were reported by their parents to have had an episode of loss of consciousness since their 11th birthday. It is easy to see why, in studies where cases are based on parental reports of seizures, high prevalence rates are

Table 1. Follow-up of children with epilepsy from the National Child Development Study (NCDS): preliminary data (June 1986)

Surveyed at:	Possible cases of epilepsy	Established epilepsy
11 years	346	64
16 years	53	16 (26 still under investigation)
23 years	99	16 (59 still under investigation)

found (Rose *et al.*, 1973). At 23 years 551 (4.4%) young people reported such an episode since their 16th birthday. Scrutiny of the questionnaires of these members of the cohort led us to suspect possible new cases of epilepsy in 152 individuals. We have so far excluded 45 of these and have confirmed epilepsy in 32, 16 new cases arising between 11 and 16 years and the same number between 16 and 23 years (Table 1). In 11 of these cases the fits had started before the 11-year follow-up but were not identified at that time (Table 2). Twenty-two of the new cases had had their first fit before the age of 16, but two of these were fit-free in the two years before the 16-year follow-up. By the age of 23 one young person had died and five of the cases had been fit-free for at least two years. In writing to the young people this year we have learned that 17 of the 32 cases have been free of fits in the last two years.

In addition to the cases of epilepsy identified from the NCDS follow-up data, we have discovered seven additional cases: five from lists made of children with

Table 2. Preliminary data on 32 individuals identified at 16 and 23 as having epilepsy (NCDS, June 1986)

	Years of age			
	By 11	By 16	By 23	By 28
No indication of epilepsy	21	8	0	0
Had/still having fits	11	20	23	9
Fit-free for 2 years or more	0	2	5	17
No information	0	2	3	5
Died	0	0	1	1
Total	32	32	32	32

Sixteen were identified from 16-year data, 16 from 23-year data.

handicap and two from scrutiny of death certificates related to the cohort. At this stage of the research we know of six deaths among 98 cases; for five of these epilepsy was recorded as the cause of death.

It is in following the natural history that consideration of epilepsy as a single entity becomes most obviously inadequate. Most studies agree in showing that children who have epilepsy alone, uncomplicated by signs of cerebral damage or other handicapping conditions, comprise about two-thirds of the child population with epilepsy; they nearly all go to ordinary school, and as they grow up show little difference from their peers in social outcomes. The present NCDS follow-up study will enable the relationships between types of epilepsy, school career and subsequent employment to be fully explored in a large, nationally representative population in which other important variables such as family background can be controlled.

Among the 64 cases identified at the 11-year follow-up, 22 were receiving special education by the age of 16. Among the 32 cases identified at the 16-year and 23-year follow-ups, and aside from the five new cases identified from lists of children with handicap, 12 had evidence of mental handicap. At 11 years no definite cause for epilepsy was found in 49 out of 64 cases, compared with 17 out of 32 later cases. In seven of the 64 children with epilepsy at 11 years there was a cause which would now be preventable. Causal factors are still being investigated in the later follow-up studies, but at least four head injuries and two other road traffic accidents have been found. A study by Ross and Bommen (1983) could find no preventable causes in 100 children seen in a district general hospital in a 12-month period.

Whereas at 11 there were slightly more boys (35) than girls (29), in common with other studies of neurological disorder in children, at age 23 there were equal numbers of young men and young women (16) among the new cases.

Analytical studies

This contribution has only given consideration to the descriptive aspects of the epidemiology of epilepsy in childhood. There is a growing body of information from analytical studies about other aspects, such as the association with psychiatric disorder considered by Rutter *et al.* (1970) in the Isle of Wight and the relationship of different types of epilepsy and drug treatment to learning and behaviour problems in children studied by Stores (1981).

CONCLUSIONS

From our understanding of the prevalence, incidence and prognosis of epilepsy, taking into account the differing types, we may both plan and evaluate local medical, educational and welfare services for children with epilepsy (Ross *et al.*, 1983). In summary: four to five per 1000 children of secondary school age have had at least two non-febrile fits, with new cases arising throughout the school years, and these can reasonably be regarded as having a history of epilepsy; about half of these children have had fits in the previous two years and can be said to have 'active' epilepsy. A further two per 1000 children have been labelled as having epilepsy but there is reasonable doubt concerning the reliability of the diagnosis. It may be expected that in a health district with a population of 250 000, there will be about 200 children of school age or below with an 'active' seizure disorder. About two-thirds of these will be in normal schools and although they may have more school absence and more learning and behaviour disorder than their peers, they will have little or no reduction in general school ability. The majority of children with epilepsy who are in special education are multiply handicapped; about one in 2000 children have intractable or very severe problems in connection with epilepsy. These children in particular require special multidisciplinary services, probably for the rest of their lives (Morgan and Kurtz, 1986). The causes of epilepsy and possibilities for prevention remain a considerable challenge.

ACKNOWLEDGEMENTS

The study is being carried out at the Institute of Child Health, London by the authors with Professor C. S. Peckham in the Department of Paediatric Epidemiology. We wish to express our gratitude to Action Research for the Crippled Child which has funded this project, based on the National Child Development Study under the aegis of the National Children's Bureau, to whom we also express our thanks.

REFERENCES

Brewis, M., Poskanzer, D. C., Rolland, C. and Miller, H. (1966) Neurological disease in an English city. *Acta Neurol. Scand.*, **24** (suppl.), 1–89.

Cooper, J. E. (1965) Epilepsy in a longitudinal study of 5000 children. *Br. Med. J.*, **1**, 1020–1022.

Crombie, D. L., Cross, K. W., Fry, J., Pinsent, R. J. F. H. and Watts, C. A. H. (1960) A survey of the epilepsies in general practice. *Br. Med. J.*, **2**, 416–422.

DHSS (1969) *People with Epilepsy—Report of a Joint Sub-Committee of the Standing Medical Advisory Committee and the Advisory Committee on the Health and Welfare of Handicapped Persons*, HMSO, London.

Goodridge, D. M. G. and Shorvon, S. D. (1983) Epileptic seizures in a population of 6000. I: Demography, diagnosis and classification, and role of the hospital services. *Br. Med. J.*, **287**, 641–644.

Gulliford, R. (1971) *Special Educational Needs*, Routledge and Kegan Paul, London.

Harrison, R. M. and Taylor, D. C. (1976) Childhood seizures: a 25-year follow-up. *Lancet*, **i**, 948–951.

Hauser, W. A. and Kurland, L. T. (1975) The epidemiology of epilepsy in Rochester, Minnesota, 1935 through 1967. *Epilepsia*, **16**, 1–66.

HOLDSWORTH, L. and WHITMORE, K. (1974) A study of children with epilepsy attending ordinary schools. I: Their seizure patterns, progress and behaviour in school. *Dev. Med. Child Neurol.*, **16**, 746–758.

KANGESU, E., MCGOWAN, M. E. L. and EDEH, J. (1984) Management of epilepsy in schools. *Arch. Dis. Child.*, **59**, 45–47.

KIORBOE, E. (1961) The prognosis of epilepsy. *Acta Psychiatr. Neurol. Scand. (suppl.)*, **150**, 166.

KURTZ, Z. (1983) Special schooling for children with epilepsy. In: *Research Progress in Epilepsy*, F. C. Rose (Ed.), Pitman Medical, Tunbridge Wells, pp. 538–546.

MILLER, D. L., ROSS, E. M., ALDERSLADE, R., BELLMAN, M. H. and RAWSON, N. S. B. (1981) Pertussis immunisation and serious neurological illness in children. *Br. Med. J.*, **282**, 1595–1599.

MORGAN, J. and KURTZ, Z. (1986) *Special Services for People with Epilepsy*, HMSO, London.

POND, D. A., BIDWELL, B. H. and STEIN, L. (1960) A survey of epilepsy in fourteen general practices. *Psychiatr. Neurol. Neurochirurg.*, **63**, 217–236.

ROSE, S. W., PENRY, J. K., MARKUSH, R. E., RADLOFF, L. A. and PUTNAM, P. L. (1973) Prevalence of epilepsy in children. *Epilepsia*, **14**, 133–152.

ROSS, E. M. and BOMMEN, M. (1983) An epilepsy clinic for children: analysis of a year's work. *Br. J. Clin. Prac. (suppl.)*, **27**, 105–108.

ROSS, E. M. and PECKHAM, C. S. (1983) Seizure disorder in the National Child Development Study. In: *Research Progress in Epilepsy*, F. C. Rose (Ed.), Pitman Medical, Tunbridge Wells, pp. 46–59.

ROSS, E. M., PECKHAM, C. S., WEST, P. B. and BUTLER, N. R. (1980) Epilepsy in childhood: findings from the National Child Development Study. *Br. Med. J.*, **1**, 207–210.

ROSS, E. M., KURTZ, Z. and PECKHAM, C. S. (1983) Children with epilepsy: Implications for the School Health Service. *Public Health*, **97**, 75–81.

RUTTER, M., TIZARD, J. and WHITMORE, K. (1970) *Education, Health and Behaviour*, Longman, London.

STORES, G. (1981) Problems of learning and behaviour and children with epilepsy. In: *Epilepsy and Psychiatry*, E. H. Reynolds and M. R. Trimble (Eds), Churchill Livingstone, Edinburgh, p. 33.

VERITY, C. M. and ROSS, E. M. (1985) Longitudinal studies of children's epilepsy. In: *Paediatric Perspectives on Epilepsy*, E. M. Ross and E. H. Reynolds (Eds), Wiley, Chichester, pp. 133–140.

DISCUSSION

Ross: The long-term development of children who have had seizures and what becomes of them as adults are vitally important questions.

Dr J. Stephenson (Glasgow): Can you expand on mortality, for which widely differing figures have been published?

Kurtz: I hope that when we have complete case identification and validation we shall have a mortality figure that can be relied on. Taylor's follow-up reported a 10% death rate by middle life (Harrison and Taylor, 1976). Our figure represents about a 5% death rate, which may or may not indicate an improvement. Virtually all reported deaths seem to have been as a result of epilepsy, which was not so in the past. The only other evidence I have is from follow-ups at a special school, where the death rates were higher, but they relate to a very handicapped population.

Epilepsy in Young People
Edited by E. Ross, D. Chadwick and R. Crawford

3

Education and epilepsy

PETER J. ROGAN
St Michael's Primary School, Knowsley, Merseyside

SUMMARY

Education of the public about epilepsy leaves much to be desired. Lack of understanding about the condition is widespread, leading to fear of epilepsy which in turn induces prejudice. A prolonged epileptic fit can be a frightening experience, but if people are educated to know what to expect then fear is reduced. Schools can play an important part here in educating the public. The Epilepsy Associations within the British Isles all run an education service, and very often a local doctor is actively involved. An authoritative viewpoint from the GP, given outside the clinic, can often open hitherto closed doors to people with epilepsy. In terms of medical education, greater priority should be given to teaching the subject of epilepsy in the medical student's curriculum.

Since the 1981 Education Act, more children with epilepsy are being integrated into mainstream schools with or without a 'statement' under the terms of the Act. A full curriculum should be available at school to children with epilepsy to develop their full range of abilities.

Education in relation to epilepsy covers three main areas: (1) medical education, (2) education of the public and (3) statutory education.

MEDICAL EDUCATION

Regarding training, I am on uncertain ground as I know very little of what goes on in medical school. However, what I do know is that those who have people with epilepsy in their families, as I do, want to believe that their doctor is an expert in the treatment of epilepsy. This leads me to speculate how much training medical students receive in the management and treatment of epilepsy. In my own field of primary education I am often asked to introduce new content into an already-crowded curriculum, and something would have to go to make way for new input. If there were to be a greater input into the medical school curriculum about epilepsy would something have to go to make room for it? And, if so, what? It is a question of priorities and, in particular, what priority should be given to the subject of epilepsy in the medical student's curriculum.

EDUCATION OF THE PUBLIC

Lack of public understanding of epilepsy causes fear, and fear in turn induces prejudice. There can be no doubt that there is a general prejudice towards those with epilepsy, not only in this country but throughout the world. In some countries epilepsy is still associated with demoniacal possession. To the general public epilepsy is still shrouded in legend and mystery. How much more tolerant would we all be if we had a little more knowledge about differing aspects of epilepsy? Being realistic I would not criticize anybody who is fearful of witnessing an epileptic seizure. I have seen hundreds and still feel afraid when the fit is prolonged. However, I know that my fear is tempered by the knowledge I have acquired about the condition.

The Epilepsy Associations operating in the UK and Ireland all run an education service. Voluntary speakers from the Associations regularly visit lay organizations to explain the nature of the condition. They advise on first-aid procedures and differing types of seizure and on educational and employment problems. Very often a local doctor is actively involved in these education programmes. Where I come from on Merseyside, we receive great support from the medical profession in our educational work.

We have to recognize that not all doctors have the time to assist in this way but maybe there are some in this audience who could offer one or two hours a year to help. The rewards are great since the authoritative viewpoint of a doctor, given outside the clinic, can open many doors to those who have epilepsy. In an audience there may be an employer who learns that epilepsy is not a bar to the type of employment he has to offer, or parents who learn that their child's seizures can be well controlled, and that he or she can grow up to enjoy a full and active life—when previously they thought that all was doom and gloom. I invite this conference to ponder as to whether the education services of the Epilepsy Associations do a valid job, and if the answer is in the affirmative, is there any help that individuals here could give?

STATUTORY EDUCATION

My working life is spent as Headteacher of a mainstream primary school in Kirkby, Merseyside. In that position I am responsible for the education of all children in our school, and we do have children with epilepsy in our care. However, not all children with epilepsy can be successfully integrated into mainstream schools, and special provision is made in three schools in Britain for those children who have specific difficulties connected with the condition. Nevertheless, since the advent of the 1981 Education Act, more and more children with epilepsy are being integrated into mainstream schools with or without a 'statement' under the terms of the Act.

In our school we have two children with epilepsy and we have learned to cope with any difficulties these may produce. All the staff need to be familiar with the condition and an essential part of their knowledge is how to administer first aid in the event of a tonic-clonic seizure. It is debatable whether this might include administration of rectal diazepam as a first-aid procedure.

I believe that the full curriculum should be available to the child with epilepsy, and swimming with adult supervision should be included as part of the physical education curriculum. However, I do have reservations about children who have such an unpredictable disorder being allowed to climb, and I do not allow this activity. Discipline exercised for the child with epilepsy should be no different to that applied to his/her peer group. Anything else would be totally unfair to all parties. I make no exceptions to this general rule.

RANGE OF ABILITIES

The intellectual abilities of epileptic children fall within the normal distribution range; some will be low attainers while others do well and go on to gain university degrees. I feel that it is essential for teachers and parents to recognize this fact so that epilepsy is not accepted as an excuse for low attainment, bearing in mind that underlying brain disorder could be the cause of low attainment as well as the epilepsy in some children.

Finally we must consider the effect on other children of having an epileptic child as a classmate. Although children can be extremely cruel to each other, correct guidance can foster caring attitudes to less fortunate classmates. In the case of epilepsy young children should clearly be taught about their own condition, and I believe there is a strong case for teaching classmates about it as well.

Publications and slide-tape programmes suited to children in different age groups and their parents can do much to inform people about epilepsy. This material is available from the Epilepsy Associations operating in Britain and Ireland.

EPILEPSY—TELL ME MORE: A SLIDE-TAPE PROGRAMME

The following extracts are taken from a slide presentation called *Epilepsy—Tell Me More* by Peter J. Rogan and illustrated by David Hollomby.

This is a story about Tommy, a ten-year-old boy who suffers from epilepsy. He lives in a town with his family and goes to the local junior school. Tommy is like many other boys; he sometimes gets into mischief and loves playing out with his friends. Occasionally he has a fit and our story tells how he learned more about his epilepsy and how his doctors helped to control the fits and his family and friends learned to be helpful . . . .

. . . Miss Jones, Tommy's teacher, brought a computer into class to help the children with their classwork. She explained that although the class computer was a wonderful machine, the computer inside the head, called the brain, was even more wonderful. However, just as the class computer sometimes goes wrong the brain can also develop little faults. We need an expert engineer to mend the class computer and an expert doctor to treat the faults in the brain.

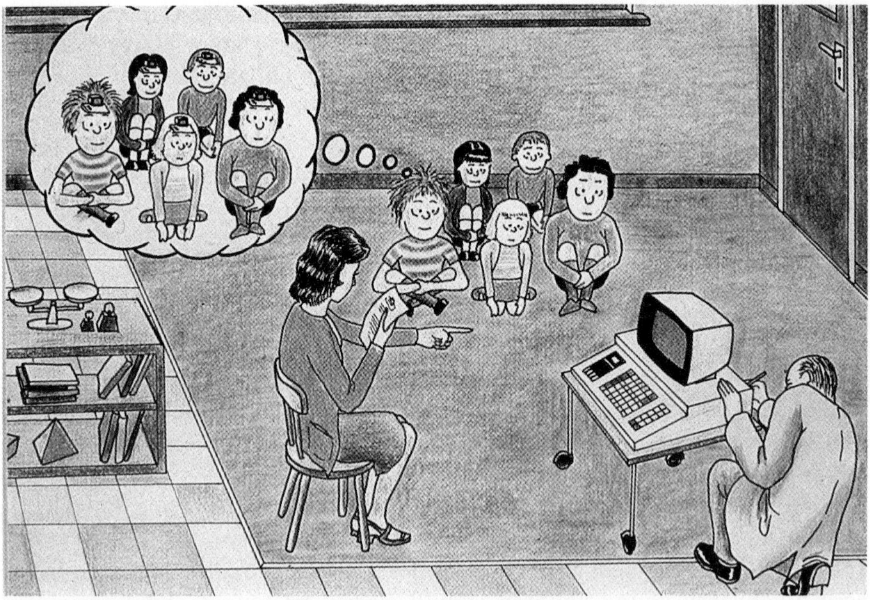

Tommy's brain had developed a fault which caused him to have one or two fits, so his Mum took him to see the family doctor. He wanted Tommy to see an expert doctor at the hospital who knew all about children's brains . . . The family doctor explained that Tommy would have to take a few hours off school to go and see the doctor at the hospital.

. . . When the big day came, he arrived at the hospital to find it very busy and he had to wait a little while before he could see the doctor.

Tommy and his Mum and Dad were asked all sorts of questions by the doctor . . . When he had finished asking the questions, the doctor told Tommy that he wanted to examine him and so the nurse helped him to get ready for the examination. The doctor listened to his chest, looked in his eyes and made lots of other tests . . .

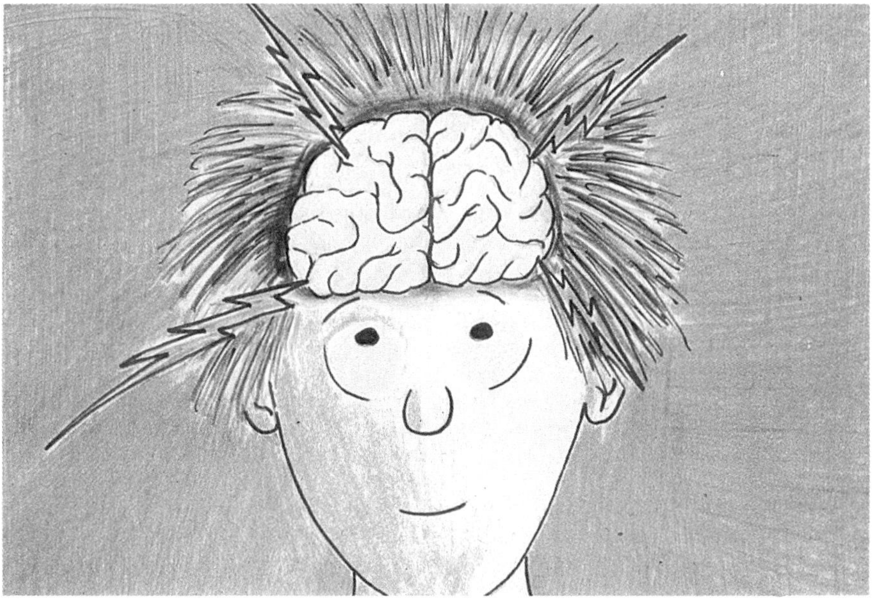

Tommy was very surprised to learn that everybody's brain gives off tiny amounts of electricity all the time, even when he or she is asleep. He was even more surprised to find that the electricity could be measured on a machine called an EEG. The doctor wanted this electricity measured because a person with epilepsy usually gives different

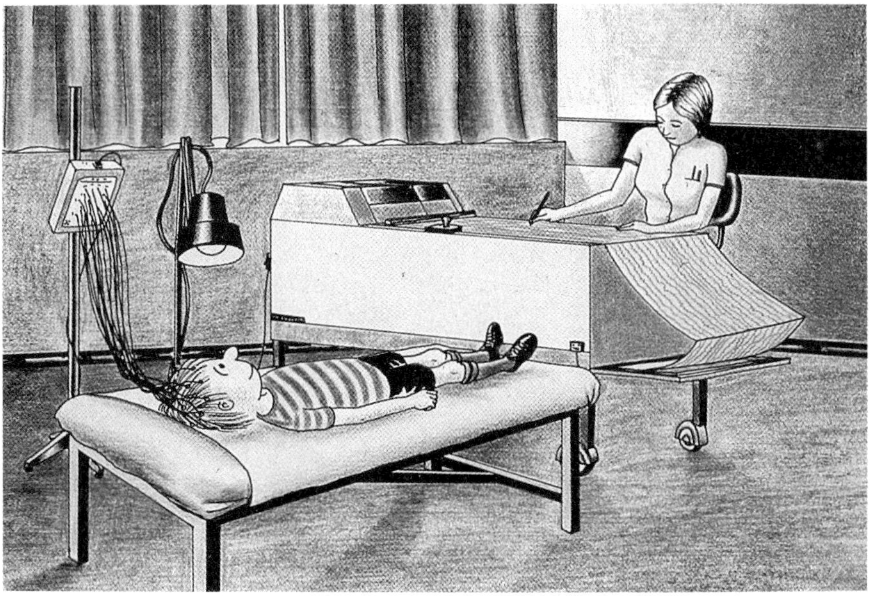

measurements from those whose brains are working as they should. The measurements can also show where the fault in the brain is to be found.

. . . At the hospital the next day, a nurse made him feel comfortable by lying him down on a bed. Little pads were fixed to his head with special glue and he was told to relax. After a while he was asked to open and close his eyes and at one time a light flashed, just like at a disco. It was all very pleasant and did not hurt even a little bit.

When it was all over the doctor looked at the patterns made on the paper by the machine and these helped him to decide that Tommy did have epilepsy. The patterns also helped the doctor to decide what type of epilepsy Tommy had. The doctor still had all the notes from the first time he met Tommy and so when he had collected all the information together he wrote to Tommy's own family doctor and told him what sort of tablets or medicine to give him.

. . . Tommy loved playing with his friends. He was as good as them at most things . . . His Dad had taught him to swim, but when he went with Tommy to the swimming baths he always asked the attendant to keep a special eye on him. Tommy never went to the baths by himself, just in case anything went wrong while he was in the water. The doctor had told Tommy that he could do almost everything that other children do, but he did not want him to ride a bicycle on busy roads and he did not want him to climb trees or anything else from which he might fall. Tommy was disappointed, but he knew himself that the doctor was right and only wanted to keep him safe and well.

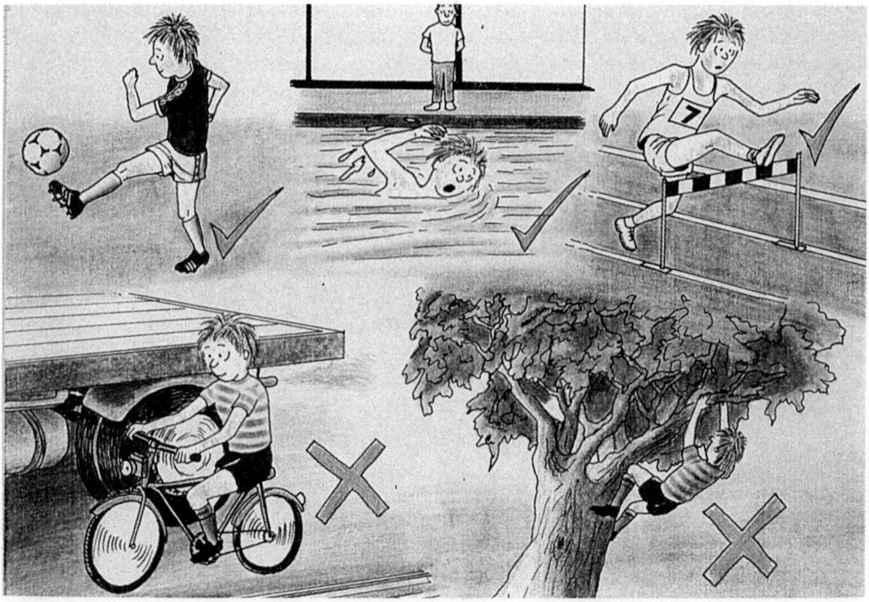

Finally the doctor had told him that the best way to keep well and enjoy all his games was to make sure he took his tablets. He was told to make a special effort never to forget to take them, because if he did he would end up having fits and miss out on all the fun.

Tommy had lots of friends and his Mum thought that they should all know what to do if he had a fit while she was not there. She wrote out a few simple instructions for them to follow . . . .

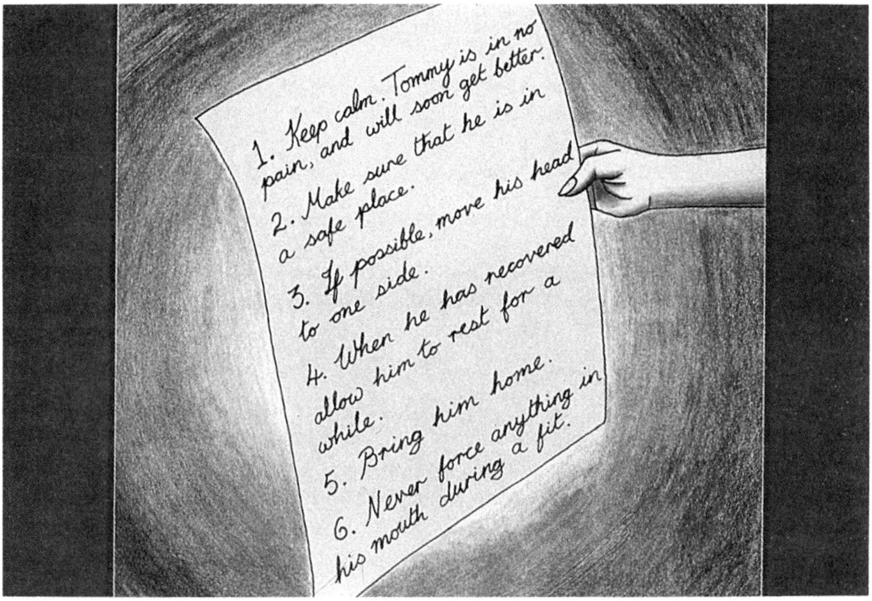
1. Keep calm. Tommy is in no pain, and will soon get better.
2. Make sure that he is in a safe place.
3. If possible, move his head to one side.
4. When he has recovered allow him to rest for a while.
5. Bring him home.
6. Never force anything in his mouth during a fit.

She also told them that very occasionally Tommy might have another fit before recovering from the first one, especially if he had forgotten to take his tablets. If this happened he would need to go to hospital in an ambulance, where doctors and nurses could look after him.

Tommy's parents went to school to see the Head and Miss Jones, his class teacher. They explained all that had been going on at the hospital and they wanted to know how he was getting on at school . . .

There was another pupil in the school with epilepsy, who was doing very well and the teachers could not see why Tommy should not do just as well, provided he was prepared to work hard.

. . . Epilepsy is nothing new or unusual. There are about one hundred thousand children in England and Wales who have epilepsy. If they were all together at the same time there would be enough children to fill Wembley Stadium . . . History tells of many famous people who have had epilepsy. You can see that if you have epilepsy you are part of a very special group of people.

Just think, it could be you who is missing from the 'Epilepsy Hall of Fame'.

FURTHER INFORMATION

British Epilepsy Association
Head Office: Anstey House, 40 Hanover Square, Leeds, LS3 1BE

Regional Offices:

Belfast	The Old Postgraduate Medical Centre, Belfast City Hospital, Lisburn Road, Belfast, BT9 7AB (Tel: 0232 248414)
Birmingham	First Floor, Guildhall Building, Navigation Street, Birmingham, B2 4BT (Tel: 021-643 7524)
Cardiff	142 Whitchurch Road, Gabalfa, Cardiff, CF4 3NA (Tel: 0222 628744)
Leeds	North Regional Centre, 313 Chapeltown Road, Leeds, LS7 3JT (Tel: 0532 621076)
London	92–94 Tooley Street, London, SE1 9SH (Tel: 01-403 4111)
Reading	72a London Street, Reading, RG1 4SD (Tel: 0734 587345)

Mersey Region Epilepsy Association, 138 The Albany, Old Hall Street, Liverpool, L3 9EY (Tel: 051-236 0990)

Epilepsy Association of Scotland, 48 Govan Road, Glasgow, G51 1JL (Tel: 041-427 4911)

Irish Epilepsy Association, 249 Crumlin Road, Dublin 12 (Tel: Dublin 557500/557017)

Epilepsy in Young People
Edited by E. Ross, D. Chadwick and R. Crawford

4

Driving and employment

JOLYON R. OXLEY
National Society for Epilepsy, Chalfont Centre for Epilepsy, Chalfont St Peter, Buckinghamshire

SUMMARY

British driving licence regulations are clear, impartial and administered by one authority, the Driving and Vehicle Licensing Centre. Employment legislation is often less specific and this allows for some flexibility of interpretation. However, the need for an accurate diagnosis is particularly important because parts of the legislation refer specifically to 'epilepsy', which is not in itself defined in law. It is therefore the physician who must carry the burden of responsibility as to what is and what is not epilepsy and decide whether the legislation is applicable to a particular case.

However, as well as barring people with epilepsy from certain types of employment, present legislation also supports the patient in providing special employment services (available to all disabled people). In practice the regulations are likely to be applied more rigorously to job applicants than to employees who develop epilepsy. Once seizures have occurred, it is essential that employees receive urgent and appropriate medical attention so that their employment prospects may be protected.

INTRODUCTION

The topics of driving and employment are aptly considered together in a book on young people with epilepsy. These activities have several features in common: both are regarded as highly desirable achievements by many, reflecting social and economic status; both are often singled out as important for the development and maintenance of self-esteem; both are affected by legislation, and both can be threatened by the advent of epilepsy. Indeed, when compiling a video programme entitled 'Attitudes' as part of an education package for social workers (Stewart *et al.*, 1987), the National Society for Epilepsy (NSE) found that the loss of a driving licence and threat to employment were identified by a group of people with epilepsy as two of the most damaging consequences of the condition.

The difficulties facing young people with epilepsy in these two areas arc based largely on other people's perception of the risk that epilepsy, or more accurately the seizure, is thought to pose to both the individual with epilepsy and to other members of society. The assessment of this risk should depend upon two factors: the likelihood of another seizure occurring in a particular individual and the consquences of such an event. The risks involved in driving have been difficult to assess accurately, partly because of a significantly high concealment rate (Taylor, 1983) and partly because of variability in clinical management. Nevertheless, it is reported that patients with epilepsy have a higher accident rate than age-matched controls (Spudis *et al.*, 1986). There have been many studies on epilepsy and employment, but only a few have looked at the problem of risk in terms of accidents at the work place. However, data indicate that those people with epilepsy who are employed are neither more accident-prone nor more likely to be absent from work than their colleagues. It remains uncertain whether these findings are unduly influenced by selective recruitment policies leading to the more disabled epilepsy sufferers being excluded. Lisle and Waldron (1986) found that employees with epilepsy are under-represented in the UK National Health Service, a very large organization, suggesting this could be the case.

Many factors influence the success or failure of a young person with epilepsy in achieving the twin objectives of driving and working. This short chapter therefore concentrates on two aspects, namely legislation and the need for accuracy in medical management.

LEGISLATION

Driving

The merits of the driving licence regulations are that they are clear, impartial and administered by one authority. The Driving and Vehicle Licensing Centre (DVLC) has its own medical staff and access to an expert medical advisory panel. The topic is extensively reviewed in *Driving and Epilepsy* (Godwin-Austen and Espir, 1983) and more recently by O'Brien (1986). The present position, following an amendment to the regulations in 1982, can be summarized as follows:

When a person with epilepsy wishes to drive for the first time the normal application form must be completed in full. A further form will be sent to the applicant requesting details about the epilepsy and information will be requested from the applicant's doctor.

A licence will be issued providing all normal requirements are fulfilled and the applicant has been completely free of fits for two years.

A licence can also be granted to an applicant who continues to have fits providing they only occur during sleep and three years have elapsed since the first fit. Applicants must also be able to drive without being likely to be a source of danger to the public for any reason.

If someone already holding a driving licence is diagnosed as having epilepsy, that person must notify the DVLC in Swansea, and stop driving until further directed by the DVLC.

A licence will not be reissued until the person fulfils the above requirement.

Re-application may be made to the DVLC after the appropriate period, at which time further medical information will be requested.

A person who has had a fit since attaining the age of five will under no circumstances be granted a heavy goods vehicle (HGV) or public service (PSV) licence. If a person holding such a licence is diagnosed as having had a seizure, the licence will be lost indefinitely.

In addition, the following points should be taken into account:

1. The regulations relate to epilepsy and, apart from the HGV and PSV rules, not a single seizure. Usually an ordinary licence will be withheld for one year following a single attack pending medical review at the end of that time.
2. Auras and epileptic myoclonic jerks are regarded as fits so far as the law is concerned and a person experiencing these during wakefulness is not permitted to drive.
3. The regulations are the same whether the person takes medication or not. Seizures that occur as a result of a change in treatment, even on medical advice, are not exempt from the regulations.
4. The regulations cannot be waived in individual cases on the grounds of the minor nature of attacks, the length of the warning period, the person never having had a fit while driving or the hardship caused by the loss of a licence.
5. Although professional driving, e.g. as a van driver or a chauffeur, is not specifically mentioned in the legislation, the medical advisory panel has consistently recommended that people with a history of epilepsy should not be employed in these capacities.

Employment

Legislation not only imposes barriers to employment for people with epilepsy but also provides special employment services which are available to all disabled people. Some jobs are prohibited to people with epilepsy on the basis of the driving licence regulations. Others are prohibited because of Act of Parliament, statutory instrument or occupational health requirements imposed by statutory bodies. Some regulations are highly specific to epilepsy such as the merchant shipping regulations but others, such as the Nurses, Midwives and Health

Visitors Act 1979 have more general health requirements which tend to exclude people who continue to have seizures. This lack of specificity can cause uncertainty but also does allow for some flexibility of interpretation. In practice, the regulations are likely to be applied more rigorously for job applicants than for employees who develop epilepsy. The overall effect of legislation on employment is summarized in Table 1, and the topic is discussed in greater detail by Craig and Oxley (1986).

Recently there has been a move to link more occupational health requirements for employees with epilepsy to the driving licence regulations (Royal College of Nursing, 1985; Brown, 1986; Betts, 1986). Although the intentions behind adopting the driving regulations as a standard of eligibility for other occupations are entirely laudable, there is a danger that people who do not fulfil these requirements, and yet have the necessary skills, might be unfairly penalized.

However, legislation is supportive as well as prohibitive. Young people with epilepsy are entitled to make use of the full range of services for disabled people provided by the Manpower Services Commission (MSC) which are reviewed elsewhere (Gloag, 1985; Edwards *et al.*, 1986). Other legislation, which is less obviously employment-related, may also assist young people with epilepsy to realize their employment ambitions. In particular, the 1981 Education Act should facilitate the early recognition of educational problems encountered by some young people and the mobilization of appropriate resources. For a more detailed consideration of this topic the reader is referred to *Epilepsy and Education* (Stores and Oxley, 1986).

Table 1. Legal barriers to employment

Seizures before 5th birthday
Train driver: London Underground
Seizures after 5th birthday
Lorry driver
Bus driver
Taxi driver
Commercial aircraft pilot
Police
Armed services
Fire brigade
Merchant navy
Seizures still occurring
Difficulties will often be encountered when working as:
Teacher in a State school
Nurse
Nursery attendant
and working:
At heights
Near water
With unguarded machines
Alone for long periods

For a number of years, sections of the disablement lobby have campaigned for specific anti-discrimination legislation, similar to that enacted for race and sex. Although there is a strong measure of support for this, the methods by which such legislation could be implemented effectively remain unclear. There has also been a trend towards encouraging better employment practices as exemplified by the MSC's Code of Good Practice on the Employment of Disabled People (Manpower Services Commission, 1984). Whether this voluntary code would be more effective if it had statutory backing remains to be seen.

MEDICAL MANAGEMENT: THE NEED FOR ACCURACY

Good medical practice for young people with epilepsy is discussed in other chapters in this book. This section concentrates on those aspects which are important for obtaining a driving licence and a job. As both these activities are affected by legislation there is a clear requirement for accuracy, particularly in the four main areas of diagnosis, treatment, counselling the individual patient, and providing information to other professionals.

Diagnosis and treatment

The need to be accurate in diagnosis may seem self-evident but it is particularly important in this context as some of the legislation refers specifically to 'epilepsy'. For example, the young adult might be barred from certain occupations (see Table 1) in error unless the nature of events occurring in childhood had been clearly established. As 'epilepsy' is a medical diagnostic label and is not defined in law, physicians must carry the burden of responsibility for deciding whether this legislation is applicable in a particular case.

The early recognition of seizures in a young person is also clearly important. This can be difficult if the attacks are non-convulsive in nature. Although their advent may prove to be a handicap, prolonged failure to recognize their true nature can lead to even greater difficulties at school, within the family and with peers. Teachers and their advisers should be fully conversant with the ways in which epilepsy can present and full use should be made of video material such as that contained in the NSE's educational package for teachers (Dowds *et al.*, 1985).

Accuracy in treatment may also be critical to the young person's career and driving ambitions. The adverse effects of an unnecessarily prolonged period of uncontrolled seizures have already been mentioned. Inappropriate treatment can add another dimension to the handicap if it causes behavioural, cognitive or cosmetic side-effects. Reliability in taking treatment can be a problem in adolescents and this may result in unnecessary seizures if the young person does not receive appropriate counselling and support. At this time a decision may be needed about withdrawing treatment if the seizures are in remission. In the light of present knowledge it seems to be easier to start treatment than to withdraw it with confidence. The results of the trial sponsored by the Medical Research Council may assist with this decision, but meanwhile the pros and cons of stopping treatment must be thoroughly discussed. Inappropriate drug withdrawal which leads to a return of seizures may well prejudice career and driving ambitions, albeit not usually irrevocably, but the damage to self-confidence and esteem can be considerable.

Guidance on careers

Medical advice may well be sought by young people with epilepsy and their families and other professionals when choosing a suitable career and job hunting. Medical guidance about careers should be based on the individual's medical details and the restrictions outlined in Table 1. Young people with continuing seizures are likely to be at a considerable disadvantage in the job market and the expertise of the specialist careers adviser for the handicapped and the Disablement Resettlement Officer may be needed. Legislation and seizures apart, employability is likely to depend substantially on educational qualifications, aptitudes and social and job-related skills. The young person with epilepsy should therefore be encouraged to take full advantage of further and higher education and training schemes operated by the Manpower Services Commission. Nevertheless, even when a career has been chosen, the actual process of applying for and starting a job may present further difficulties. Completing application forms, explaining the epilepsy at interview and coping with seizures at work, all require young people with epilepsy to be confident, reassuring and knowledgeable about their own epilepsy. The need for comprehensive patient education about epilepsy cannot therefore be over-emphasized. Many, however, feel that to declare epilepsy on an application form is a sure way of being rejected without an interview. Nevertheless, concealment of the epilepsy may well lead to dismissal (if a seizure occurs at work) without recourse to an industrial tribunal due to infringement of the Health and Safety at Work Act (1974). However, the recommendations recently proposed for a Code of Good Practice covering recruitment and health disclosure (Floyd and Espir, 1986) would go a long way to helping young job applicants with epilepsy. The main elements of this proposed code are:

1. All job application forms should be accompanied by explanatory notes indicating the health standards required.
2. No questions about health and disabilities should be included in job application forms.
3. Health declaration forms should only be inspected after the candidates have been selected and only by an occupational health physician or those delegated and qualified to do so.

4. Rejection on health grounds should be possible only after a medical examination.

Support at work

The sudden advent of seizures can be devastating if employment is threatened because of concern over safety at work, loss of driving licence or simple prejudice. It is essential that this does not happen as a result of medical mismanagement. Once seizures have occurred, however, it is also essential that employees receive accurate medical attention as a matter of urgency, in order that their employment prospects should be protected. A number of professionals, including the general practitioner, the hospital specialist and the occupational health physician, may be needed to support someone with epilepsy at work. This task is greatly assisted by close liaison between the professionals and by easy exchange of information and opinion.

With adequate support the majority of young people with epilepsy will progress satisfactorily so far as employment is concerned, but some, particularly those with uncontrolled seizures or who have other handicaps, may remain rather vulnerable. Such people may have problems not only in securing and keeping a job but also in achieving promotion. However, the temptation simply to blame the epilepsy must be resisted as other factors such as performance and personality may be highly relevant.

REFERENCES

BETTS, T. A. (1986) Employees with epilepsy in the National Health Service. *Br. Med. J.*, **292**, 764–765.

BROWN, I. (1986) Developing guidelines for epilepsy at work—The occupational physician's role. In: *Epilepsy and Employment—A Medical Symposium on Current Problems and Best Practices*, F. Edwards *et al.* (Eds), Royal Society of Medicine, London, 53–58.

CRAIG, A. and OXLEY, J. (1986) Statutory and non-statutory barriers to the employment of people with epilepsy. In: *Epilepsy and Employment—A Medical Symposium on Current Problems and Best Practices*, F. Edwards *et al.* (Eds), Royal Society of Medicine, London, 21–31.

DOWDS, C., CRAIG, A. G. and OXLEY, J. (1985) *An Educational Package for Teachers.* National Society for Epilepsy, Chalfont St Peter.

EDWARDS, F., ESPIR, M. L. and OXLEY, J. (1986) *Epilepsy and Employment—A Medical Symposium on Current Problems and Best Practices*, Royal Society of Medicine, London.

FLOYD, M. and ESPIR, M. L. (1986) Assessment of medical fitness for employment: The case for a code of good practice. *Lancet*, **ii**, 207–208.

GLOAG, D. (1985) Occupational rehabilitation and return to work: I. General services. *Br. Med. J.*, **290**, 1135–1138.

GODWIN-AUSTEN, R. B. and ESPIR, M. L. (1983) *Driving and Epilepsy—and Other Causes of Impaired Consciousness*, Royal Society of Medicine, London.

LISLE, J. R. and WALDRON, H. A. (1986) Employees with epilepsy in the National Health Service. *Br. Med. J.*, **292**, 305–306.

Manpower Services Commission (1984) *Code of Good Practice on the Employment of Disabled People*. MSC, Sheffield.

O'BRIEN, S. J. (1986) The controversy surrounding epilepsy and driving—a review. *Public Health*, **100**, 21–27.

Royal College of Nursing (1985) *Health Screening of Entrants for Nurse Training*. Report of the Working Party of the Royal College of Nursing/Society of Occupational Health Nursing. RCN, London.

SPUDIS, E. V., PENRY, J. K. and GIBSON, P. (1986) Driving impairment caused by episodic brain dysfunction. *Arch. Neurol.*, **43**, 558–564.

STEWART, P., DOWDS, C., CRAIG, A. G. and OXLEY, J. (1987) *Epilepsy: An Educational package for Social Workers*, National Society for Epilepsy, Chalfont St Peter (in press).

STORES, G. and OXLEY, J. (1986) *Epilepsy and Education—A Medical Symposium*, Medical Tribune Group, London.

TAYLOR, J. (1983) Epilepsy and other causes of collapse at the wheel. In: *Driving and Epilepsy—and Other Causes of Impaired Consciousness*, R. B. Godwin-Austen and M. L. E. Espir (Eds), Royal Society of Medicine, London, pp. 5–7.

Epilepsy in Young People
Edited by E. Ross, D. Chadwick and R. Crawford

5

Personal relationships

LEONARD THORNTON
Department of Child and Adolescent Psychiatry,
Royal Manchester Children's Hospital

SUMMARY

The young person with epilepsy frequently experiences difficulties in psychosocial functioning, particularly in the field of interpersonal relationships. However, such handicaps may present to the physician only in the form of poorly controlled seizures, non-compliance with treatment or changes in behaviour and symptom patterns. As a result, these difficulties may pass undetected, or be inappropriately treated.

Awareness of adolescent development and of the effects of seizure disorder on this process are necessary for understanding the predicament of the young person with epilepsy. Early detection of underlying problems is facilitated by the use of specific screening questions relating to mood state, life events, family and social functioning. Appropriate management of the individual depends on the presence of good liaison between the various disciplines involved.

INTRODUCTION

The growth of consultation-liaison psychiatry in recent years has been prompted by increasing awareness of the psychological accompaniments to chronic physical disorders, and the need for an integrated approach to treatment. Within this group of disorders, the young person with epilepsy is particularly burdened by psychosocial difficulties, and their handicaps are not always related to the severity of the seizure disorder. Studies of adolescents with epilepsy (Richardson and Friedman, 1974; Freeman *et al.*, 1984; Dorenbaum *et al.*, 1985) show several problem areas including absence of friendships, difficulties with family and existing peer-group relationships, social maladjustment (particularly at school), poor self-confidence and depressive feelings.

Psychological dysfunction can persist into adult life. Emotional and interpersonal issues are prevalent concerns of adults with epilepsy (Dodrill *et al.*, 1984). The relatively low marriage rates among people with epilepsy (Dansky *et al.*, 1980) suggests persisting difficulties in forming and maintaining stable close relationships. Among those with epilepsy who marry, subsequent relationship breakdown is associated with poorer emotional adjustment. They are found to be more pessimistic about their life and to use repression and denial mechanisms more often to cope with stresses (Batzel and Dodrill, 1984). Early detection and management of psychosocial problems is therefore essential if later handicap is to be avoided.

THE LANGUAGE OF DISTRESS

The medical outpatient clinic is an important meeting place where patients and their families can express their concerns. However, the clinic setting encourages the presentation of problems in a medically-framed language and the attribution of these difficulties to physical causes. Hence, poorly-controlled seizures, somatic symptoms and medication are the matters that doctor and patient tend to discuss.

Parents of the adolescent with epilepsy will report behaviour problems. These tend to be disruptive in nature and are therefore socially visible. The presence of depression, on the other hand, although handicapping, is less frequently noticed by parents. It is therefore less spontaneously 'offered' to the doctor for treatment. Somatic symptoms, overt behavioural disturbance, social withdrawal and failure to comply with treatment are all powerful channels through which young people may express their emotional distress. However, if the physician restricts his area of enquiry, focuses down prematurely on initial presentation and seeks to understand these features only in terms of physical pathology, then the psychological meaning behind the symptoms will remain masked. Underlying many of these cases are major interactive issues which are the real handicap. An understanding of the overall 'predicament' of the adolescent with epilepsy is therefore required (Taylor, 1982).

DEVELOPMENT AND IDENTITY

An accurate assessment of the young person's social functioning requires an awareness of the developmental expectations and stresses which occur in adolescence. This is a time of rapid development, and successful negotiation of this stage sees the individual achieve a more permanent inner image of self. The development of autonomy, self-esteem and social skills are central to the formation of a mature identity. These processes allow the individual to attain independence from the family, form intimate relationships, establish a work role and function within society as an adult.

The handicaps generated by 'being epileptic' can severely impede normal development. If the disorder has been present since childhood, the individual is particularly vulnerable. Failure of early development is a poor preparation for coping with the tasks of adolescence. If the burden of epilepsy has been insuperable normal personality development does not occur, producing in adolescence a state of identity confusion. Alternatively the only sense of self and role which the individual may possess is that of the sick person, with epilepsy as a 'career'. This may appear to be the only lifestyle available.

FAMILY ISSUES

The impact of seizure disorder can produce major changes within family relationships. Major or minor readjustments may be made in an attempt to deal with the actual and anticipated handicaps of the young person with epilepsy. In response to their anxieties about the child, parents may become overprotective. In some cases, this reflects an overcompensated reaction to initial parental rejection. Such ambivalence may rear its head in later years where parental overconcern is tinged with thinly-disguised hostility directed towards the teenager with epilepsy who has chronically burdened them.

Certain parental attitudes are associated with impaired academic and social adjustment in the young person with epilepsy (Hartlage and Green, 1972). The ability to take initiative and to develop acceptable expressions of one's emotions and sexuality are particularly required in adulthood. However, parental overprotection and suppression of the individual does not allow the opportunity to experiment and acquire such skills. Similarly, the lowered expectations held by parents (Long and Moore, 1979) reinforce poor self-esteem, further compounding the situation. The shy, immature and socially inept teenager reflects these early rearing practices.

Reciprocal overdependency on parents is a particularly marked response in young people with epilepsy (Hartlage *et al.*, 1972; Stores, 1978; Hoare, 1984a). The anxious attachment present in the parent-child relationship fails to allow the natural formation of autonomy and separation.

School refusal is a frequent presentation of separation anxiety in childhood and adolescence. However, the persistence of attachment disorder into young adulthood is a neglected phenomenon. Reluctance to attend college and work may be present, or fear of leaving home to live independently, but these separation problems are again masked by more clinically noticeable features. Labels such as 'agoraphobia' or 'anxiety state' may be given to such cases, but unfortunately they convey little or no information about the core of long-standing difficulties which give rise to the symptoms.

Within the family, the individual's function can become restricted. In response to the unpredictability of epilepsy, families tend to adopt a rigid, autocratic hierarchy (Ritchie, 1981). Such a family system can protect itself against the disruptive effects of the disorder and allow efficient problem-solving to take place. However, as a result, the young person with epilepsy becomes excluded from active participation in this process and may withdraw entirely from family interactions.

The young person's life is thereby controlled by others and the opportunity to develop decision-making and interpersonal skills is stifled. Higher rates of marital breakdown (Sillanpää, 1973), and of maternal and sibling psychiatric disturbance (Hoare, 1984b) have all been reported in families where there is a child with epilepsy. This may reflect the decompensation of coping mechanisms in family members living in a chronically stressed home.

However, in being identified as the sick family member, the person with epilepsy is at risk of becoming the symptom bearer and scapegoat for the underlying family pathology. In such cases, psychological management of the individual alone will therefore prove insufficient.

BEING DIFFERENT AND FACING STRESS

The need to conform and identify with one's peer group is an important feature of adolescence. During this time, comparison with friends becomes increasingly the mechanism for evaluating self-image and confirming separateness from parents.

The sudden loss of normality experienced following the onset of epilepsy in this age group can produce reactions akin to those experienced in bereavement. By comparison, the young person with long-standing epilepsy may have had effectively no experience of being normal (Taylor, 1969). However, the increasing social pressures of adolescence rekindle the awareness that they are different from their peers.

Unlike physical handicaps that are always visible, epilepsy evokes little support from the community. People with epilepsy are a particularly stigmatized group. The seizure speaks up unannounced in a dramatic manner and cares not for social etiquette. The fear of loss of control in public sets in motion defensive manoeuvres of secrecy and withdrawal. These are particularly marked if the individual has been sensitized by prior ridicule and rejection from his peer group. Such defences may initially protect an already fragile self-esteem, but in the longer term socially isolate the individual.

The ability to understand and accept the real limitations imposed by epilepsy is necessary if emotional maturity is to be achieved. At a time of rapidly developing independence, the adolescent finds himself shackled with unwanted restrictions and a dependence on adults, hospitals and tablets. Failure to accept the disorder as being part of self is reflected by the attempts of the individual to reject and deny its presence. For example, the responsibility for the management of the disorder may be handed back to the parents. The twenty-year-old who still relies on mother to give him his anticonvulsants, arrange hospital appointments and speak up for him at the clinic has failed to adapt to his handicap. 'It's not my epilepsy, it's really my mum's' is his message. Mother has also played her part in maintaining the situation, and so to an extent has the doctor.

Non-compliance with treatment is a common feature in the teenager with epilepsy. It can reflect a basic misunderstanding of the need for medication. However, it also indicates a powerful attempt to deny and break away from the predicament of having epilepsy.

To facilitate adjustment, early intervention in the form of counselling and further support as required is essential for the individual and the parents. Inappropriate dependence and overprotection should be actively discouraged.

The limited experience and restricted field of activity make changes in the social universe of the young person with epilepsy particularly stressful. Leaving school, job interviews, starting work and even pleasurable social events can all be regarded as threatening. Recent life events are associated with the presentation of recurrent somatic complaints in teenagers (Greene *et al.*, 1985), and may induce an increase in seizure frequency. They also appear to play a role in precipitating the onset of psychiatric disorder in childhood and adolescence (Goodyer *et al.*, 1985). The impact which these life events have on the individual should therefore not be underestimated.

ASSESSMENT AND LIAISON

Screening for the presence of psychosocial difficulties in the clinic is an important complement to the traditional medical procedures. However, assessment of the individual's functioning based primarily on parental interview and a perfunctory chat with the adolescent is to be discouraged. This occurs particularly in long-standing cases where the established practice has been for the parents, usually mother, to bring the child to the clinic and for the transfer of information to be between doctor and parent(s). Parental information alone provides an incomplete picture. However, reported behaviour and symptoms which are situation specific, for example, aggressive outbursts occurring only at home, should suggest the presence of interactive factors, and further enquiry is warranted.

An individual interview with the adolescent is essential. It acknowledges his or her separate identity and conveys the message that personal views and concerns are sought and will be taken seriously. The teenager is the sole provider of information regarding his inner thoughts, mood state and accounts of peer-group relationships. Enquiries should be made about daily life. What are his or her roles and responsibilities at home? What are his relationships like with other family members? Can he seek appropriate help and advice from the family if he has a problem? What difficulties are encountered at school or work? Does he have close friends in whom he can confide? Does a wider network of acquaintances exist? How is leisure-time spent? Are his pursuits solitary or do they involve making social contacts?

Changes in seizure frequency, symptom pattern and behaviour should prompt enquiries about recent and imminent life events, plus the individual's feelings about the threat which they hold. The presence of low self-opinion and recent social withdrawal should alert the physician to the presence of a depressive disorder and the risk of suicide in this group should be borne in mind.

Adolescents at individual interview express a higher rate of affective symptoms compared with parental reports (Rutter *et al.*, 1976). Specific questions relating to mood state, depressive thoughts and associated disturbances of sleep, appetite and concentration are therefore required. The concerns of the parents are not necessarily the same as those of the adolescent. The individual's appreciation of seizure disorder, management and related personal anxieties, for example, about employment, marriage and having children, all need exploration. This permits clarification and correction of any existing misconceptions. Such information requires regular updating to keep pace with the individual's needs and developmental level. The explanations given to the nine-year-old will not suffice for the 17-year-old.

In the presence of powerful situational and personal variables, alterations in anticonvulsant medication alone will be of limited value in the attempts to treat the individual. The drug regimen should be critically evaluated and consideration given to the role of complementary therapeutic approaches (Taylor and McKinlay, 1984).

Following assessment, psychiatric referral may be considered appropriate, e.g. where the presence of psychiatric disorder, handicapping psychosocial dysfunction or disturbed family relationships is suspected. The need for such a referral should be discussed in the first instance with the liaison-psychiatrist.

Regular liaison meetings between the psychiatrist and the medical team facilitate the understanding of the problems encountered by the physician and the underlying psychological processes involved. As a result, the psychiatric referral system is utilized more appropriately and joint management of cases can develop. The success of psychiatric intervention depends on the individual and family member's psychological awareness. Motivation is enhanced by prior explanation of the reasons for referral, the possible role of psychological factors in current difficulties and the need for further specialist assessment.

Individual psychological treatments may include counselling, social skills training, cognitive therapy and brief focal psychotherapy. Where major interactive difficulties exist within the home, a family therapy approach may be indicated (Goodyer, 1986).

In view of the several professional agencies often involved in the overall management of the individual, therapeutic approaches may overlap or even be contradictory. It is therefore important that efficient channels of communication exist between all the professionals involved. The multidisciplinary case conference is the most appropriate format for the formulation and monitoring of an integrated treatment plan. Such professional relationships are necessary if the predicament of the young person with epilepsy is to be understood and ultimately relieved.

REFERENCES

BATZEL, L. W. and DODRILL, C. B. (1984) Neuropsychological and emotional correlates of marital status and ability to live independently in individuals with epilepsy. *Epilepsia*, **25**, 594–598.

DANSKY, L. V., ANDERMANN, E. and ANDERMANN, F. (1980) Marriage and fertility in epileptic patients. *Epilepsia*, **21**, 261–271.

DODRILL, C. B., BREYER, D. N., DIAMOND, M. B., DUBRINSKY, B. L. and GEARY, B. B. (1984) Psychosocial problems among adults with epilepsy. *Epilepsia*, **25**, 168–175.

DORENBAUM, D., CAPPELLI, M. C., KEENE, D. and MCGRATH, P. J. (1985) Use of a child behavior checklist in the psychosocial assessment of children with epilepsy. *Clin. Pediatr. (Phila.)*, **24**, 634–637.

FREEMAN, J. M., JACOBS, J., VINING, E. and RABIN, C. E. (1984) Epilepsy and the inner city schools: A school-based program that makes a difference. *Epilepsia*, **25**, 438–442.

GOODYER, I. M. (1986) Family therapy and the handicapped child. *Dev. Med. Child Neurol.*, **28** 247–250.

GOODYER, I. M., KOLVIN, I. and GATZANIS, S. (1985) Recent undesirable life events and psychiatric disorder in childhood and adolescence. *Br. J. Psychiatry*, **147**, 517–523.

GREENE, J. W., WALKER, L. S., HICKSON, G. and THOMPSON, J. (1985) Stressful life events and somatic complaints in adolescents. *Pediatrics*, **75**, 19–22.

HARTLAGE, L. C. and GREEN, J. B. (1972) The relation of parental attitudes to academic and social achievement in epileptic children. *Epilepsia*, **13**, 21–26.

HARTLAGE, L. C., GREEN, J. B. and OFFUTT, L. (1972) Dependency in epileptic children. *Epilepsia*, **13**, 27–30.

HOARE, P. (1984a) Does illness foster dependency? A study of epileptic and diabetic children. *Dev. Med. Child Neurol.*, **26**, 20–24.

HOARE, P. (1984b) Psychiatric disturbance in the families of epileptic children. *Dev. Med. Child Neurol.*, **26**, 14–19.

LONG, C. G. and MOORE, J. R. (1979) Parental expectations for their epileptic children. *J. Child Psychol. Psychiatry*, **20**, 299–312.

RICHARDSON, D. W. and FRIEDMAN, S. B. (1974) Psychosocial problems of the adolescent patient with epilepsy. *Clin. Pediatr. (Phila.)*, **13**, 121–126.

RITCHIE, K. (1981) Research note: interaction in the families of epileptic children. *J. Child Psychol. Psychiatry*, **22**, 65–71.

RUTTER, M., GRAHAM, P., CHADWICK, O. F. D. and YULE, W. (1976) Adolescent turmoil: fact or fiction? *J. Child Psychol. Psychiatry*, **17**, 35–56.

SILLANPÄÄ, M. (1973) Medico-social prognosis of children with epilepsy. *Acta Paediatr. Scand.*, suppl., **237**.

STORES, G. (1978) Schoolchildren with epilepsy at risk for learning and behaviour problems. *Dev. Med. Child Neurol.*, **20**, 502–508.

TAYLOR, D. C. (1969) Some psychiatric aspects of epilepsy. In: *Current Problems in Neuropsychiatry*, R. N. Herrington (Ed.), Headley Bros, Ashford, pp. 106–109.

TAYLOR, D. C. (1982) Epilepsy: a model of sickness. In: *Psychopharmacology of Anticonvulsants*, M. Sandler (Ed.), Oxford University Press, New York, pp. 129–135.

TAYLOR, D. C. and MCKINLAY, I. (1984) When not to treat epilepsy with drugs. *Dev. Med. Child Neurol.*, **26**, 822–827.

PANEL DISCUSSION

Dr. R. C. Adams (Newport, IOW): Perhaps I could draw the audience's attention to a report from Manchester in last week's BMJ about the interviewing techniques of young doctors, which revealed three very important things (Maguire *et al.*, 1986a and b). One is that techniques in interviewing are established in the very early years of practice. The report goes on to show a significant difference in doctors' ability to recognize psychiatric morbidity in their patients when they have had psychiatric training, especially with video feedback. And the third finding, which is very disturbing, is that all doctors are bad at imparting information to their patients. There is clearly scope for improvement here—and in appraising the effects of epilepsy. Some years ago we had a student in the children's department who had developed epilepsy since starting at medical school. At this point he had been strongly discouraged from continuing his training and told that he probably would not be able to get a job. As a patient, I wouldn't like my surgeon to have epilepsy, but I really don't see why my neurologist shouldn't.

Dr L. Thornton (Manchester): It is important that medical students should receive training in interview techniques which can be learned very quickly. I was involved in the earlier Manchester work as a group tutor. Training comprised four weekly group sessions with the students, each lasting about an hour and involving feedback and interpretation of their recorded interviews with patients. Interviewing skills improved quite dramatically and appeared to be maintained. The imparting of information is absolutely essential. We find that many adolescents understand little about their seizure disorder. This is not because the paediatrician has not told them, but because he has not checked that the patient has actually understood. Many myths about epilepsy build up from this lack of understanding.

Dr E. M. Ross (London), Chairman: At the University of Kingston in Canada, there is a special department for teaching interview and examination skills, where volunteer patients (often retired people) with genuine complaints come up and spend half a day each week. Particularly for students at the beginning of their clinical period, this seems an exceedingly good idea.

Professor C. R. B. Joyce (Basle): About 15 years ago I was rather deeply involved in medical education, and it is sad to realize that nothing much has changed since. There are a lot of good ideas, like those just mentioned, but they seldom seem to be carried into practice. Again and again, one has the impression not so much that the wheel is being reinvented as that people are discovering the need for somebody to invent it. How can we increase the likelihood that the excellent ideas that do exist will actually be carried into practice *across the board*, not just locally by those who have the enthusiasm and research interest?

Dr M. R. Trimble (London): What evidence is there that Napoleon had epilepsy? Several other examples chosen in Mr Rogan's booklet are questionable too: Van Gogh became psychotic and the later paintings became very stylized, obsessional and repetitive. He was not a typical epilepsy patient, and of course Julius Caesar just didn't make very many friends.

Mr P. J. Rogan (Knowsley): The evidence for Napoleon's epilepsy comes from a standard text on the history of epilepsy, 'The Falling Sickness' by Owsei Tempkin (Johns Hopkins Press), but I gather that this view is not universally accepted.

Dr J. R. Oxley (National Society for Epilepsy): As regards doctors and other NHS employees with epilepsy, I'm not aware of any statutory health criteria for doctors. Indeed, several doctors who continue to have seizures are practising physicians in this country, and no doubt there are others worldwide. The problem with extending something like the driving licence regulations to NHS employees is that trained staff who are doing their jobs perfectly well might then be at risk of dismissal. Clear-cut regulations have advantages, but may put individuals' employment in jeopardy unnecessarily. There is also a danger that restrictive regulations might be extended to jobs where a seizure would pose no real risk to anyone. The accurate assessment of risk in the workplace is difficult and input from a knowledgeable occupational health physician is essential.

Dr J. Stephenson (Glasgow): Why is it that people with anoxic seizures due to abrupt excessive vagal activity don't seem to attract either the stigmata of epilepsy or the legal bars? It might be helpful if we could see what separates them from the various forms of epilepsy.

Oxley: The so-called stigmata identified by surveys suggest that people's stereotypes of epilepsy are partly dependent on their having seen somebody having a seizure and more particularly on associated handicaps. They have rather little to do with the epilepsy *per se*. Other handicaps and overt seizures tend to mould stereotypes.

Dr J. Corbett (East Grinstead): As regards what children should be allowed to do, my knowledge is mainly of children with severe learning disorders, living within the community and going to school. While it's true that most of those who died in childhood did so as a result of their epilepsy, one must allow these children the dignity of risk. They need to be able to lead as normal a life as possible. The staff working in special schools therefore need quite a lot of help to come to terms with the fact that some children with severe neurological disorders are going to die during their school careers. We know there is a risk, for example, if a seizure occurs while swimming. But do we know how many accidents are attributed to people with epilepsy driving?

Oxley: In a series reported by Taylor (1983) of accidents due to collapse at the wheel investigated by the police in which the driver survived, 38% were due to generalized seizures. Seventy per cent of these people had not declared their condition to the DVLC, and 12% were having their first fit. Other studies reviewed recently (Spudis *et al.*, 1986) have suggested that people with epilepsy in general have higher accident rates than age-matched controls. However, these authors also point out the enormous methodological difficulties in collecting accurate information.

Dr P. Heaton (Paddington Green, London): If one is trying to educate a potential employer about the possible hazards of employing someone who suffers from epilepsy, it's important to be able to give them a truthful picture of the impact that the individual's epilepsy is likely to have on his work. Have there been any studies of individuals with epilepsy in the absence of other handicaps, in which accidents at work and absenteeism have been quantified?

Oxley: Yes. One of the most notable in this country was the study done in the British Steel industry by Dasgupta *et al.* (1982). The problem is of course that the study population may not be typical of people with epilepsy as a whole. Those people with epilepsy who are in employment have accident and sickness rates that are probably no higher than for other employees, but this may be because people with less well-controlled epilepsy who might have more accidents and/or be absent more often are less likely to be employed. The situation may be clarified by a proposed study in the Civil Service, which has a very positive approach to employing people with epilepsy. There has also been a proposal to do a similar parallel study of employees with epilepsy in the National Health Service.

Ross: It would be useful if all of us made great efforts to ensure that the occupational health physicians who work in hospitals are abreast of current thinking on employment of people with epilepsy, many of whom apply for NHS work.

Dr S. D. Shorvon (London): To what extent do employers have a right to medical information? I endorse the suggestion that job application forms should not ask for medical details and that the appointment should be subject to medical examination. Responsibility for assessing the medical handicap is thus handed over to the doctor by the employer or interviewing committee, who may not have any medical knowledge.

Oxley: People with epilepsy should have a right, like any job applicant, that any information they give about themselves is handled and analysed by somebody qualified to do so. Legally however, the employer has an absolute right to employ or not to employ, whatever any doctor says. The requirement to disclose medical information is largely governed by the Health and Safety at Work Act of 1974, which lays obligations both on the employer and on the job applicant or employee. The employer has to disclose hazards in the workplace that might prejudice the health and safety of workers, and the employee is under an obligation to disclose any health problem that might put him at risk. If he wilfully conceals that information, he can be dismissed without recourse to an industrial tribunal.

Dr D. W. Chadwick (Liverpool): What do you advise a young person, applying for a job for which he is adequately qualified, who is faced with a first application form that demands medical information, which seems likely to be used by someone who is not medically qualified?

Oxley: Knowingly and wilfully failing to disclose epilepsy when specifically asked for it on an application form invites problems in the future. What we should all seek to do, reflecting what Simon Shorvon has said, is to try to encourage employers and the Institute of Personnel Managers and everybody else concerned to separate medical details from the information which is purely related to the job. The medical history can then be disclosed in the confidence that it will be screened by somebody who knows how to assess it. Meanwhile I recommend that job applicants certainly do not lie when filling in forms. One young person with epilepsy I know only discloses the epilepsy at interview, by which time he has usually got the job because he has the right qualifications, experience and personality.

Rogan: I have sometimes had difficulties with doctors who have actually advised parents not to inform the school of the child's epilepsy. Although doctors have difficulties about betraying confidences, it is a gross disservice to the child and to the parents and the teacher if the doctor actively encourages parents to withhold information. Then the first we know of a child's epilepsy is the child writhing around on the floor.

Dr R. W. Newton (Manchester): As regards responsibility for the epileptic child in school, do you consider that an action could be brought against a 'locum' parent—either a care attendant in a hostel or a teacher at school—for withholding rectal diazepam?

Rogan: I would be willing to give rectal diazepam to a child who was in danger, but I have two difficulties. First, somebody would have to teach me, and second, I certainly would not give rectal diazepam to a female pupil by myself. We would have to take somebody out of a class to assist, there is a danger of possible litigation, and I cannot see my colleagues in the teaching profession readily accepting this responsibility.

Dr Y. F. Ransley (Epsom): I entirely agree with you. In ordinary schools, I don't think rectal diazepam should be given by teachers. Moreover, children with epilepsy who go to normal schools should't have to take their routine drugs at school. The same applies to many conditions.

Rogan: I would go as far as administering any drug which had to be taken during the lunch break. This is relatively rare, but the occasion sometimes arises, for example, when a child is fit for school after five days though his course of treatment is not yet completed.

Ross: Is there any antiepileptic drug that has to be taken more often than six-hourly? No? Then there is no need to take these drugs to school.

Dr A. S. Ahuja (Wigan): However, asthmatics do need to take Ventolin and sodium cromoglycate in school; PE teachers often give this medication, and I see no reason why that should not continue.

Dr M. Noronha (Manchester): In your guidance to teachers and parents, Mr Rogan, could you ask them to record what happens during a fit and the circumstances in which it occurs?

Rogan: Yes. Some parents may have difficulty in expressing themselves clearly, but there is certainly a case, where a child has a seizure at school, for the teacher to document exactly what has happened and to pass that report to the school health service.

Dr J. Stephenson (Glasgow): In a normal school, the most common first fit is a fainting fit in late childhood or early adolescence, not an epileptic seizure. If it's being called epilepsy by the time the child reaches hospital, the quickest way to solve the problem is to phone up the school and ask the teachers what happened.

REFERENCES

DASGUPTA, A. K., SAUNDERS, M. and DICK, D. J. (1982) Epilepsy in the British Steel Corporation: an evaluation of sickness, accident and work records. *Br. J. Ind. Med.*, **39**, 145–148.

MAGUIRE, P., FAIRBAIRN, S. and FLETCHER, C. (1986a) Consultation skills of young doctors: I. Benefits of feedback training in interviewing as students persist. *Br. Med. J.*, **292**, 1573–1576.

MAGUIRE, P., FAIRBAIRN, S. and FLETCHER, C. (1986b) Consultation skills of young doctors: II. Most young doctors are bad at giving information. *Br. Med. J.*, **292**, 1576–1578.

SPUDIS, E. V., PENRY, J. K. and GIBSON, P. (1986) Driving impairment caused by episodic brain dysfunction. *Arch. Neurol.*, **43**, 558–564.

TAYLOR, J. F. (1983) Epilepsy and other causes of collapse at the wheel. In: *Driving and Epilepsy—and other Causes of Impaired Consciousness*, R. B. Godwin-Austen and M. L. E. Espir (Eds), Royal Society of Medicine International Congress and Symposium Series, No. 60, Royal Society of Medicine, London, pp. 5–7.

Section II: Therapies

Epilepsy in Young People
Edited by E. Ross, D. Chadwick and R. Crawford

6

When should anticonvulsant treatment be started?

SIMON SHORVON
Institute of Neurology and National Hospital, Queen Square London, and Chalfont Centre for Epilepsy, Chalfont St Peter, Buckinghamshire

SUMMARY

In deciding whether to initiate anticonvulsant treatment it is essential to establish the diagnosis of epilepsy and to classify the seizure type. Such a label given to a patient may necessitate regular medication for long periods, and it may carry serious medical, psychological and social repercussions. Syncopal or psychogenic attacks can be mistaken for epileptic attacks, and their differential features need to be understood. If the patient has long-standing symptoms or a marked personality disorder, then the diagnosis may call for skilled specialist assessment.

The risk of seizure recurrence with and without treatment needs to be estimated. Recurrence is more likely if the first attack was recent, and treatment recommendations should therefore take into account the period of time since the initial seizure. Recurrence risks vary in different clinical settings, and a careful clinical evaluation is crucial in the decision to initiate treatment. The precipitating factors, the seizure characteristics, personal and social factors, and the risks of toxicity due to anticonvulsant drugs need also to be taken into account.

INTRODUCTION

The decision to treat seizures with anticonvulsant drugs is a major event in a young person's life. It may be the final confirmation of the diagnosis of epilepsy, it may mean regular medication for long periods, and it may have serious medical, psychological and social repercussions. While this decision is

Table 1. Questions to consider when deciding whether to initiate anticonvulsant treatment in a previously untreated patient

Is the diagnosis certain?
What are the risks of recurrence of seizures without treatment?
What are the risks of recurrence of seizures with treatment?
Are any precipitating factors relevant?
Are the seizure characteristics relevant?
Are personal factors relevant?
What are the risks of side-effects to treatment?

straightforward in many cases, in a minority—perhaps 20%—it may be difficult to decide whether treatment is appropriate, and this may depend on a number of factors, some of which are complex and ill-defined. The knee-jerk reaction of advising drug treatment after two seizures, in disregard of any other factors, is to be deprecated. In all cases counselling is imperative concerning the role of treatment, the length of time it will be continued, its effectiveness and its drawbacks. Furthermore, the new patient may only just have received a diagnosis of epilepsy, and may need time to adjust to this as well as to the prospects for treatment. Table 1 lists some of the aspects which should be accounted for before starting drug therapy, and these are briefly discussed below.

THE DIAGNOSIS OF EPILEPSY

The diagnosis of epilepsy should be certain before treatment is started. In the adolescent and young adult, the differential diagnosis of epileptic seizures is relatively easy—probably easier than in young children or in mature adults—and problems arise mainly with syncopal or psychogenic attacks. Both are not infrequently mistaken for epileptic attacks, so that patients may be misdiagnosed and consequently mistreated over a considerable period. Syncope, for instance, was the final diagnosis in more than one-third of new cases of possible epilepsy referred for EEG in Gastaut's laboratory (Gastaut, 1974). Reflex syncope is especially common in young female patients, and is a far more common cause of blackouts or 'funny turns' than epilepsy. Table 2 lists some features which help differentiate syncope from epileptic attacks; none are absolute, but in most cases differentiation should be straightforward. Cardiac syncope precipitated by cardiac arrhythmia is also relatively common in the young due to congenital cardiac disease, and a careful cardiac evaluation should always be made in a young patient presenting with episodic symptoms.

Psychogenic attacks present a particular problem in adolescent female patients and are more common than generally appreciated. The diagnosis is often easily made, although in exceptional cases (particularly in patients with long-standing

Table 2. Features helpful in the differentiation of epileptic seizures and reflex syncope

Feature	Epileptic seizure	Syncope
Precipitant	Unusual	Commonly an emotional, painful or stressful event
Circumstances	Any	Usually upright posture. Crowded, hot surroundings or emotional, stressful situation
Onset	Usually abrupt. May be short aura	May be gradual, feeling of faintness, nausea, greying of vision, sweating, hotness
Motor phenomenon	Often tonic or tonic-clonic. Clonic movements often prominent with characteristic amplitude and frequency	Usually flaccid, with no movements. May be short tonic spasm. May be a few clonic jerks, but usually brief, unco-ordinated and of low amplitude
Skin colour	May be pale or flushed	Pale
Respiration	Stertorous, foaming	Shallow, slow
Incontinence	Common	Rare
Tongue biting	Common	Rare
Vomiting	Unusual	Often
Injury	Common	Rare
Postictal	Often drowsy, confusion, sleep	Usually nil
Duration of unconsciousness	Often minutes	Usually 10 seconds or so

symptoms and a marked personality disturbance) it may require skilled and specialized assessment. Features which help to differentiate epileptic and psychogenic seizures are listed in Table 3, though none of these is pathognomonic. It should also be remembered that the two types of attack may co-exist in the same patient.

If the diagnosis is uncertain, it should be kept under review and will usually become clear with the passage of time. In routine practice there is almost no place for a 'trial of treatment' in a suspected but unconfirmed case, as the evaluation of such a trial is almost invariably inconclusive. Tentative treatment always complicates assessment, and inevitably lengthens the time taken to make a firm diagnosis.

The diagnosis of epilepsy should include a classification of seizure type and an assessment of aetiology, and these too may influence the requirement for treatment.

Table 3. Features helpful in differentiating between convulsive psychogenic and convulsive epileptic seizures

Feature	Epileptic seizure	Psychogenic seizure
Precipitant	Usually none	Often an emotional precipitant
Circumstances:		
in sleep	Common	Rare
when alone	Common	Less common
Prodroma	Rare	Common
Onset	Usually abrupt. May have short aura	May be gradual with increasing emotional symptoms
Cry at onset	Common	Unusual
Vocalization	During automatism	Common during seizure
Motor phenomenon	Stereotyped. Usually both tonic and clonic phase. Clonic movements slow as seizure continues	Variable. Often tonic or clonic only. Clonic components vary in amplitude and frequency during the attack. Pelvic thrusting. Pseudo-clonic movements
Injury	Common	Rare
Incontinence	Common	Unusual
Tongue biting	Common	Rare
Consciousness	Usually totally lost in convulsive seizures	Variable, often possible to communicate during an attack
Restraint	No effect	May resist, sometimes terminates an attack
Duration of convulsion	Usually short	May be prolonged
Termination of attack	Usually short (but with automatism sometimes). Confusion common. Drowsiness or sleep common	May be gradual, often with emotional display. Confusion unusual. Drowsiness or sleep unusual

RISKS OF SEIZURE RECURRENCE (WITH OR WITHOUT TREATMENT)

It may seem obvious that because treatment is given to lessen the chance of seizure recurrence, some estimate of untreated risk of recurrence needs to be made. Unfortunately, there is little agreement about these risks, and such estimates as there are have varied widely, depending on the population studied, the method of data collection and the criteria for entry to the study (Shorvon, 1984). After a first isolated seizure, estimates of recurrence have ranged from 27% to 82% (Table 4). The higher figures have usually been noted in

Table 4. Studies of the recurrence rates of seizures after a first single attack

	n	Patient selection	Follow-up* (months)	Recurrence† (%)
Thomas (1959)	48	Cases referred to an EEG department	ns	27
Johnson *et al.* (1972)	77	Young adult males,	6	34
		naval recruits (excluding	12	49
		organic causes, alcohol,	24	57
		drug abuse)	36	58
Saunders and Marshall (1975)	33	Referrals to an EEG department	10–48	33
Hauser and Kurland (1975)	769	Community based survey of Rochester, Minn. (including recurrent provoked seizures as single seizures)	24	67
Cleland *et al.* (1981)	70	Adult referrals to a neurology clinic with untreated 'major' seizures (excluding head injury, drug overdose)	3–120	39
Hauser *et al.* (1982)	244	Hospital referrals with 'unprovoked seizures'	12	16
		(including multiple seizures on a single	24	21
		day, excluding acute symptomatic fits)	36	27
Goodridge and Shorvon (1983b)	114	General practice based survey of Tonbridge, Kent (all seizures regardless of aetiology)	36	82
Elwes *et al.* (1985)	133	Referrals from a hospital	1	20
		casualty department with	3	32
		tonic-clonic seizures	12	62
			36	71

* Period of follow-up after first seizure.
† Percentage of patients having a second seizure during the specified follow-up period.

community-based or prospective studies, and are more representative of an unselected population than are the studies from hospital records or EEG departments. In all studies, the risks of recurrence are greatest in the days or weeks after the first attack (as was noted by Gowers 100 years ago); in about 30% of cases, the second attack will have occurred within three months of the first, and in about three-quarters of cases within two years. Thus, the recommendations for treatment should take into account the period which has elapsed since the first seizure.

After two or more attacks, the risks of recurrence are higher, but data in this area are more sparse. Most patients in whom a diagnosis is made are treated at this stage, and because of this, there is little information about the course of the untreated condition. If the attacks are widely spaced treatment is often withheld, although there is no agreement about how far apart the seizures should be. It is certainly true, however, that the more infrequent the seizures, the less likely the subsequent recurrence.

On treatment, most patients suffer only a small total number of attacks. For instance in one community-based survey of non-febrile seizures, more than half the patients with firmly diagnosed epileptic seizures had less than ten attacks in all (Goodridge and Shorvon, 1983a and b). How far treatment is responsible for this good prognosis is unclear, and there is some evidence to suggest that if treatment is delayed, the ultimate prognosis may be worsened (Shorvon and Reynolds, 1982; Reynolds *et al.*, 1983). If this is so, the case for early effective treatment becomes overwhelming, but further research is required on this point (Shorvon *et al.*, 1985).

Epileptic seizures occur in a variety of clinical settings, and recurrence risks of course are influenced by various clinical factors (Table 5). A high risk of recurrence is associated, for instance, with structural cerebral disorders, spike-wave or frequent focal spiking on EEG recording, partial seizures, abnormal neurological signs, mental retardation or handicap. A careful clinical evaluation is crucial in the decision to initiate treatment.

There have been no adequate studies of the effectiveness of therapy after a single attack, and authoritative advice cannot be given on this point. Several

Table 5. Features associated with an increased risk of seizure recurrence in epilepsy

Certain seizure types (e.g. partial seizures, tonic seizures, absence seizures, etc.)
High previous seizure frequency
Long duration of epilepsy
Structural or diffuse cerebral disorders
Certain epileptic syndromes (e.g. primary generalized epilepsy, Lennox-Gastaut syndrome, etc.)
Additional neurological or psychiatric handicap
Intellectual deficit
No immediate precipitant

investigations of initial treatment have been performed in drug-naive patients after two or more seizures, however, which show that monotherapy with an appropriate first-line anticonvulsant drug will provide complete seizure control in between 50 and 90% of cases; the use of serum level monitoring to control dosage where necessary further improves this outcome (Shorvon, 1984).

PRECIPITATING FACTORS

In a minority of cases of epilepsy, the seizures may have a well-defined precipitant (Table 6). In adolescents, alcohol or drug abuse, fatigue, lack of sleep and/or menstruation are the commonest precipitating factors. Photosensitivity is seen particularly in primary generalized epilepsy, and in myoclonic seizures, and is more common in the young person with epilepsy. Fever in older children may also precipitate seizures, but the specific syndrome of *febrile convulsions* has a distinct prognosis and needs to be considered separately.

It makes obvious sense to advise the patient to avoid situations known to precipitate seizures. Nevertheless, in most cases, the decision to treat should be made irrespective of such precipitating factors, as it is rare for seizures to occur exclusively in their presence. Alcohol-induced seizures are an exception, and it is often sufficient simply to recommend total abstinence without the need for anticonvulsant medication.

SEIZURE CHARACTERISTICS

The conventional view of the role of anticonvulsant treatment is that it alleviates the symptoms, namely the seizures, of epilepsy (rather than being curative); the nature of the symptoms should therefore be an important factor in considering treatment in any individual case. The following three main features need to be assessed.

Type of seizure

Patients with occasional brief minor attacks which do not interfere with normal activities may not require treatment, although this is often an individual decision.

Table 6. Common precipitating factors for seizures in young patients

Fever	Menstrual cycle
Stress	Photic stimulation
Fatigue	Alcohol
Sleep disturbance	Drug abuse

Timing of the seizures

Similarly, patients with only occasional nocturnal seizures may well prefer not to receive medication, even if the attacks are generalized convulsions. However, it should be remembered that in many such cases, diurnal seizures will develop (Janz, 1974).

Frequency of seizures

If the seizures are very infrequent, treatment should probably be postponed. How long the period between seizures should be to allow therapy to be deferred is an arbitrary question, however, and there are few data concerning these time-related aspects of seizure recurrence.

Before withholding therapy in active epilepsy, however, it should be remembered that seizure type and frequency may change, that early treatment may not only suppress seizures, but may also prevent the evolution of the condition to chronic epilepsy, and that epileptic seizures themselves may result in serious injury or death.

PERSONAL FACTORS

Attitude to epilepsy and treatment

It is vital to counsel all patients carefully about their epilepsy and its treatment, as misconceptions, resentment or ignorance may worsen the seizures and compromise treatment. Good compliance is essential for successful therapy, but it will not be achieved unless the patient fully accepts the need for treatment and understands its role in a realistic fashion. The prescription of long-term anticonvulsant therapy without explanation will often fail, and may lead to hostility and loss of trust.

Social factors

The activities and aspirations of the patient may also be important factors in the decision to start therapy. These are individual matters, and should be considered in all patients before initiating treatment. Areas of importance include schooling, leisure activities and employment. A balance should be struck between the psychological and domestic implications of treatment and of seizures. In adolescence, the question of driving is often a major issue, although it is advisable to warn a young person who has developed seizures that driving may well be compromised in the future by any recurrence, and the patient's future domestic or employment plans should take this into account.

TOXIC SIDE-EFFECTS

If anticonvulsant therapy were entirely innocuous, then the decision to initiate therapy would be easy. Unfortunately, treatment has side-effects (Woodbury *et al.*, 1982) which may be serious and even fatal, and the decision to treat should be taken in the light of these risks. For the purposes of this contribution, the toxic side-effects may be conveniently considered in the following five groups.

Acute idiosyncratic reactions

These occur with all presently used anticonvulsant drugs, are often minor (e.g. rash) and resolve when the drug is discontinued. Occasionally, more severe reactions occur, and these may be life-threatening or even fatal. For instance, worldwide at least 60 deaths due to acute hepatic failure have occurred on valproate therapy, 17 cases of acute hypersensitivity to phenobarbitone, 13 deaths due to aplastic anaemia on carbamazepine therapy and six deaths on ethosuximide. Other severe hypersensitivity reactions may occur including acute pancreatitis on valproate and severe dermatological reactions on phenytoin or carbamazepine.

Acute dose-related side-effects (intoxication)

Most anticonvulsant drugs at high doses will reliably produce encephalopathic symptoms, which usually resolve when the dose is reduced. Patients should be warned about these effects, but they should not usually influence the decision to treat.

Side-effects on starting therapy

Many drugs produce mild encephalopathic or gastrointestinal effects soon after starting therapy. These effects usually recede spontaneously. The patient should be warned in advance of this risk and the dose built up gradually to minimize it. Again this should not usually influence the decision to treat.

Chronic (non-dose-related) side-effects

The chronic toxicity of anticonvulsant drugs has received considerable attention in recent years (Reynolds, 1975), and is of concern to both patients and physicians. The frequency of such effects increases with prolonged therapy, with high dosage and with polytherapy. The chronic side-effects usually have more influence on the choice of drug than the decision to treat, but patients should be given information about these potential risks. Many of the toxic effects are minor and many cause no obvious symptoms. In choosing treatment for the young patient the most important are the encephalopathic and cosmetic effects. The benzodiazepine and barbiturate drugs in particular may cause depression, sedation or behavioural changes. Similar effects are seen less frequently with phenytoin and valproate, and carbamazepine seems the least likely of the major anticonvulsants to produce mental changes. Cosmetic effects such as facial coarsening, hirsutism and gum hypertrophy are common on phenytoin therapy, and may also occur on treatment with phenobarbitone. Valproate causes weight gain in a significant proportion of patients, and may also result in hair loss or curling. These cosmetic effects may be a particularly important consideration in adolescence.

Teratogenicity

Anticonvulsant treatment is associated with an approximately three-fold increase in fetal malformation. These effects vary with individual drugs. Phenytoin, for instance, may cause facial clefts, congenital cardiac defects, and other dysmorphic effects, and valproate may result in neural tube defects. Absolute risks have proved difficult to estimate, and it has been impossible to disentangle the deleterious effects of either seizure activity or genetic influences on the fetus from those of the anticonvulsant drugs. How these risks should affect the decision to treat is controversial. If anticonvulsant treatment can be safety delayed until after the first trimester this may be advisable in some cases, although evidence that it lessens the teratogenic risks in women with epilepsy is lacking. Again, these effects will more frequently influence the choice of drugs rather than the decision to treat.

REFERENCES

Cleland, P. G., Mosquera, I., Steward, W. P. and Foster, J. B. (1981) Prognosis of isolated seizures in adult life. *Br. Med. J.*, **283**, 1364.

Elwes, R. D. C., Chesterman, M. B. and Reynolds, E. H. (1985) Prognosis after a first untreated tonic-clonic seizure. *Lancet*, **ii**, 752–753.

Gastaut, H. (1974) Syncopes: generalised anoxic cerebral seizures. In: *Handbook of Clinical Neurology*, vol. 15, P. J. Vinken and G. W. Bruyn (Eds), North Holland, Amsterdam, pp. 815–835.

Goodridge, D. M. G. and Shorvon, S. D. (1983a) Epileptic seizures in a population of 6000. 1: Demography, diagnosis and classification, and the role of the hospital services. *Br. Med. J.*, **287**, 641–644.

Goodridge, D. M. G. and Shorvon, S. D. (1983b) Epileptic seizures in a population of 6000. 2: Treatment and prognosis. *Br. Med. J.*, **287**, 645–647.

Hauser, W. A. and Kurland, L. T. (1975) The epidemiology of epilepsy in Rochester, Minnesota 1935 through 1967. *Epilepsia*, **16**, 1–66.

HAUSER, W. A., ANDERSON, V. E., LOEWENSON, R. B. and MCROBERTS, S. M. (1982) Seizure recurrence after a first unprovoked seizure. *N. Engl. J. Med.*, **307**, 522–528.

JANZ, D. (1974) Epilepsy and the sleeping-waking cycle. In: *Handbook of Clinical Neurology*, vol. 15, P. J. Vinken and G. W. Bruyn (Eds), North Holland, Amsterdam, pp. 457–490.

JOHNSON, L. C., DE BOLT, W. L., LONG, M. T., ROSS, J. J., SASSIN, J. F., ARTHUR, R. J. and WALTER, R. D. (1972) Diagnostic factors in adult males following initial seizures. *Arch. Neurol.*, **27**, 193–197.

REYNOLDS, E. H. (1975) Chronic toxicity of anticonvulsant drugs. *Epilepsia*, **16**, 319–352.

REYNOLDS, E. H., ELWES, R. D. C. and SHORVON, S. D. (1983) Why does epilepsy become intractable? *Lancet*, **ii**, 952–954.

SAUNDERS, M. and MARSHALL, C. (1975) Isolated seizures: an EEG and clinical assessment. *Epilepsia*, **16**, 731–733.

SHORVON, S. D. (1984) The temporal aspects of prognosis in epilepsy. *J. Neurol. Neurosurg. Psychiatry*, **47**, 1157–1165.

SHORVON, S. D. and REYNOLDS, E. H. (1982) Early prognosis of epilepsy. *Br. Med. J.*, **285**, 1699–1701.

SHORVON, S. D., ESPIR, M. L. E., STEINER, T. J., DELLAPORTAS, C. I. and ROSE, F. C. (1985) Is there a place for placebo-controlled trials of antiepileptic drugs? *Br. Med. J.*, **281**, 1328–1329.

THOMAS, M. H. (1959) The single seizure: its study and management. *JAMA*, **169**, 457–459.

WOODBURY, D. M., PENRY, J. K. and PIPPENGER, C. E. (1982) *Antiepileptic Drugs*, Raven Press, New York.

DISCUSSION

Dr W. H. Schutt (Bristol): Giving reliable information to your patient may provoke anxiety about possible serious side-effects. How do you get over this?

Shorvon: Patients sometimes ask 'What are the serious side-effects of these drugs?' I think one is then obliged to put the risk in context: millions of prescriptions with a small number of hepatic reactions, for instance. If side-effects are not mentioned and then develop subsequently, the patient may stop taking the drug.

Dr E. M. Ross (London): In the last few years, alternative or unorthodox practitioners have also been looking after some patients with epilepsy. This is of course all part of the current reaction against powerful drugs, and I feel if we are to be credible we must counter this by taking people into our confidence and giving them as much information as possible about the actions and side-effects of drugs.

Shorvon: I personally have no objection to people trying different types of alternative medicine, providing the alternative practitioners don't interfere with the medical treatment at the same time.

Dr R. McWilliam (Stirling): Do you think ultimately it should be for the patient and/or his parents to make the decision about treatment? If you simply present them with the various advantages and disadvantages, if it's their own decision, perhaps they will be more likely to cooperate.

Shorvon: Patients require authoritative advice as well as information, and I think should be given one's own view of whether treatment is necessary. Obviously, in the final analysis it's up to the patient to decide whether to take a drug. Although patients should be involved, a lot of people come to the doctor for a decision.

Epilepsy in Young People
Edited by E. Ross, D. Chadwick and R. Crawford

7

Social implications of drug treatment and withdrawal

DAVID CHADWICK
Walton Hospital, Liverpool

SUMMARY

What are the factors which govern the decision to withdraw antiepileptic therapy in the young? Most paediatricians and neurologists would advocate giving antiepileptic drugs until such time as the patient has been free from seizures for more than two years. Withdrawal of medication should then be gradual but relapse occurs in 20–40% of patients. Most relapses occur within six months of reducing dosage. Primary generalized seizures, i.e. absence and tonic-clonic seizures, have been reported by some authors to have a more favourable prognostic significance than partial seizures. Factors which may be important to a good prognosis are a normal EEG before withdrawal, a history of few tonic-clonic seizures, and young age at onset of epilepsy.

INTRODUCTION

Clinicians have reasonably clear and uniform ideas concerning the factors which influence the decision to initiate therapy for epilepsy, but the decision to discontinue therapy is based on less common ground. Most paediatricians and adult neurologists would agree that antiepileptic drugs should be prescribed until such time as patients have been seizure-free for two or more years. While as many as 80% of patients who develop seizure disorders are likely to achieve such remissions, usually early in the course of therapy (Annegers *et al.*, 1979), clinicians remain uncertain whether remission represents 'cure' of that patient's epilepsy or 'control' dependent on continued antiepileptic therapy.

This differentiation obviously has immense practical importance to decision making but is also one of great importance to patients. Many patients feel that freedom from the stigma of epilepsy will only be removed satisfactorily once seizures have ceased *and* treatment is no longer necessary.

The decision to undertake a trial of antiepileptic drug withdrawal is one that must be made by patients and their families following advice from the clinician, rather than by the clinician alone. This is necessary because of the social implications of the decision. Patients are being asked to make judgements of the relative risks of continued drug taking against the risks of further seizures inherent in drug withdrawal. There can be no doubt that the social pressures and difficulties of this decision are greatly increased as patients with epilepsy pass from their school years into full adult life. This is reflected by the fact that patients seen by paediatricians are most likely to be advised to discontinue therapy after a two-year remission, while those seen by an adult neurologist are more likely to be advised to continue the therapy.

MEDICAL FACTORS

A few studies have been undertaken to determine the success of withdrawing anticonvulsant drugs and the factors that identify patients likely to remain free of seizures. These studies and their results have been reviewed elsewhere (Chadwick, 1985; Chadwick and Reynolds, 1985). Comparison is difficult because there is often little information about the patients, a lack of uniformity in length of remission before withdrawal of antiepileptic drugs, and often no information about the period of withdrawal and the duration of follow-up. Estimates tend to be crude figures after follow-up for an arbitrary period.

However, some broad measure of agreement emerges. The risk of relapse for children in remission is about 20% overall, whereas relapses in series which have included adults are approximately 40%. Most relapses occur during or within six months of dose reduction. This information is of limited value to patients as they require some estimate of their own individual risk of relapse. While a number of factors may influence the risk of relapse, offering an individual prognosis is difficult at present. There is some general agreement that the more severe and long-lasting a patient's active epilepsy before remission the greater the risk of relapse.

Seizure classification may be of some help though this remains controversial. Primary generalized seizures (both absence and tonic-clonic seizures) have been reported by some authors to have a favourable prognostic significance compared to partial seizures, but other authors have disagreed with this. The presence of neuropsychiatric handicap or cerebral pathology affects prognosis adversely. Whether electroencephalography is helpful is again controversial. Certainly only those EEGs taken after a period of remission are likely to be of value. In children there seems little doubt that the presence of persisting EEG abnormalities influences prognosis adversely, but whether this is true in adults also remains uncertain.

Emerson *et al.* (1981) assessed the relative contribution of several factors to the prognosis after withdrawal of drugs. They found that a normal EEG before withdrawal and a history of only a few tonic-clonic seizures were of greatest importance. Thurston *et al.* (1982), again in children, found that the most important adverse factors were: long duration of epilepsy, the presence of focal motor seizures, or combinations of seizure types, and the presence of neurological deficit. Shinnar *et al.* (1985) found that the EEG, seizure type and age of onset were the major determinants of outcome.

Patients must set the risks of continued therapy against those of drug withdrawal. Unfortunately, these are even more difficult to quantify. Usually patients who enter remission do so on small doses of antiepileptic drugs which are unlikely to carry a high long-term risk of chronic toxicity. However, it is now recognized that many drugs do have subtle effects on cognition and behaviour even at therapeutic dosage (Reynolds, 1983), and their discontinuation may well be beneficial to some patients. Ultimately the patient's own feelings about taking medication become of great importance.

Patients must also consider the risk of having seizures even when therapy is continued. It is assumed that they are more likely to have seizures when they stop taking antiepileptic drugs than when they continue taking them. Advice to continue drugs indefinitely does not, however, guarantee continued remission, partly because patients may become less compliant. Unfortunately, there is no information available to compare the rate of relapse in patients randomly allocated to continued therapy or withdrawal. Such information is needed because it might help to answer the most important question of all: to what extent does stopping treatment increase the risk of further seizures?

Surprisingly, we lack any data that satisfactorily describe the risk of relapse after two or three years' remission in patients continuing treatment. Annegers *et al.* (1979) found a seizure risk of 1.6% a year in patients remaining free of seizures for five years. The risk of relapse might, however, be greater in patients who have attained shorter remissions, and indeed the study of Elwes *et al.* (1984) suggests that the risk of subsequent relapses may be as high as 8% a year after a two-year remission. Thus the benefits of continued antiepileptic treatment in terms of better control of seizures might not be great enough to outweigh the adverse effects, particularly if poor compliance is a problem in patients advised to continue treatment.

OTHER PROBLEMS

Unsolved problems include the question of whether increasingly long periods free of seizures carry a better prognosis for discontinuing treatment. Unfortunately, there is no information about whether withdrawal of antiepileptic drugs is considered best after two, three, five, or more years of remission.

Data permitting assessment of the importance of the relative speed at which antiepileptic drugs are withdrawn are also limited. All clinicians are aware of the dangers of suddenly stopping treatment, and all studies agree that relapses commonly occur during or shortly after a reduction in treatment or total withdrawal. Oller-Daurella *et al.* (1976) found that withdrawing drugs very slowly resulted in a much lower risk of relapse than that reported in other studies including adult patients.

Do seizures arising in close association with withdrawal of drugs suggest a continuing epileptic disorder that requires continued treatment? Or can they be regarded simply as withdrawal seizures similar to those that occur in otherwise non-epileptic subjects following withdrawal of regular treatment with shorter-acting sedative drugs such as alcohol, barbiturates and benzodiazepines? The latter would of course not necessarily demand reintroduction of treatment.

SOCIAL FACTORS

It is clear from the above that it is difficult to give firm advice and predictions to patients and their families. In these circumstances social factors become important in decision-making.

The vast majority of children with epilepsy are educated in 'mainstream' schools. Here they undoubtedly benefit from involvement in a wide range of activities which are important in the development of social skills. Unfortunately, this kind of integration often ceases when the child leaves school. While his friends may successfully go on to find employment, this will often be more difficult for a young person with a history of epilepsy. All too often a vicious circle of social isolation and reduced expectations becomes established. Too many individuals become dependent on a small family group and have few contacts outside it. For these reasons, making the correct decision about continued antiepileptic therapy becomes of crucial importance, and ideally trials of drug withdrawal should take place before school-leaving age. After this time a number of factors may influence decision-making.

EMPLOYMENT

The young person with a history of epilepsy is more likely to find difficulty gaining satisfactory employment than his peers. Continued remission of epilepsy greatly increases the chance of getting a job, and this will usually act as a pressure to continue therapy. However, on rare occasions the contrary may be true. The author is aware of employers who have made an offer of employment that was conditional on an individual being off his medication!

DRIVING

At the age of 17 a young person with a history of epilepsy can gain a provisional driving licence as long as there has been either freedom from seizures altogether for a period of two years, or only nocturnal seizures for a period of three years. Once a person has gained a driving licence its possession is a potent argument for continued therapy, as any seizures occurring on drug withdrawal will inevitably lead to the loss of that licence for a minimum two-year period. The loss of such a licence may secondarily affect employment. These regulations are undoubtedly the most common reason for patients maintaining their therapy after a period of remission, and their severity may to some extent be seen as a constraint on a patient's freedom of choice.

LEISURE PURSUITS

The young person with epilepsy often enjoys participation in activities that may be viewed as 'risky' if a seizure were to occur while participating. These include swimming, cycling and horse riding, all of which can be undertaken satisfactorily subject to a few commonsense precautions and responsible supervision. However, such pursuits may become regarded as unacceptable and too risky during a period of antiepileptic drug withdrawal.

REPRODUCTION

Concerns about the way in which drug therapy may affect contraception and pregnancy, and vice-versa, are very real to young women with a history of epilepsy. The fact that drugs which act as enzyme-inducers (phenobarbitone, phenytoin, and carbamazepine) may all reduce the efficacy of oral contraceptive agents and necessitate the use of higher dose oestrogen preparations may be seen by many patients as an indication for considering withdrawal of antiepileptic drugs. A much more potent argument, however, is the risk of teratogenicity associated with drug therapy. Most young women contemplating pregnancy who have been seizure-free for approximately two years would see this as a reason for undertaking a trial of antiepileptic drug withdrawal before pregnancy.

Finally, there is the overall concern young people have that a recurrence of seizures may interfere with their abilities to undertake an independent existence. Although some people may be able to accept the risk of seizures while they are living at home with their family, this risk may become much less acceptable once they have moved away from the family home and are living independently.

CONCLUSIONS

The factors which influence decision-making about the withdrawal of antiepileptic drugs are summarized in Table 1. Current practice is based on

Table 1. Criteria for stopping antiepileptic treatment

Absolute requirement	Factors in favour	Factors against
Two to three years free of all seizures	Childhood epilepsy	Late onset epilepsy
Patient's informed agreement	Primary generalized epilepsy	Partial epilepsy
	Absence of cerebral disorder	Cerebral disorder
	Short duration of epilepsy	Long duration of epilepsy
	Normal electro-encephalogram	Abnormal electro-encephalogram
	Non-driver	Driver

inadequate clinical information, and this increases the weight that must be placed on social factors. It is to be hoped that our ability to identify those patients with low and high risks of relapse following antiepileptic drug withdrawal will be increased by a large prospective study of antiepileptic drug withdrawal now being undertaken on a multicentre basis in the United Kingdom and Europe.

REFERENCES

ANNEGERS, J. F., HAUSER, W. A. and ELVERBACK, L. R. (1979) Remission of seizures and relapse in patients with epilepsy. *Epilepsia*, **20**, 729–737.

CHADWICK, D. (1985) The discontinuation of antiepileptic therapy. In: *Recent Advances in Epilepsy*, vol. 2, B. M. Meldrum and T. A. Pedley (Eds), Churchill Livingstone, Edinburgh, pp. 111–124.

CHADWICK, D. and REYNOLDS, E. H. (1985) When do epileptic patients need treatment? Starting and stopping medication. *Br. Med. J.*, **290**, 1885–1888.

ELWES, R. D. C., JOHNSON, A. L., SHORVON, S. D. and REYNOLDS, E. H. (1984) The prognosis for seizure control in newly diagnosed epilepsy. *N. Engl. J. Med.*, **311** 944–947.

EMERSON, R., D'SOUZA, B. J., VINING, E. P., HOLDEN, K. R., MELLITS, E. D. and FREEMAN, J. M. (1981) Stopping medication in children with epilepsy. *N. Engl. J. Med.*, **304**, 1125–1129.

OLLER-DAURELLA, L., PAMIES, R. and OLLER, L. (1976) Reduction or discontinuance of antiepileptic drugs in patients seizure free for more than five years. In: *Epileptology*, D. Janz (Ed.), Thieme, Stuttgart, pp. 218–227.

REYNOLDS, E. H. (1983) Mental effects of antiepileptic medication: a review. *Epilepsia*, **24** (Suppl. 2), S85–S95.

SHINNAR, S., VINING, E. P. G., MELLITS, E. D., D'SOUZA, B. J., HOLDEN, K., BAUMGARDNER, R. A. and FREEMAN, J. M. (1985) Discontinuing antiepileptic medication in children with epilepsy after two years without seizures. *N. Engl. J. Med.*, **313**, 976–980.

THURSTON, J. H., THURSTON, D. L., HIXON, B. B. and KELLER, A. J. (1982) Prognosis in childhood epilepsy. *N. Engl. J. Med.*, **306**, 831–836.

DISCUSSION

Dr R. McWilliam (Stirling): One of the most important and useful developments in childhood epilepsy in recent years has been an attempt to categorize or classify children under headings of epileptic syndromes based on seizure type, EEG appearances, and the history of the child's neurological examinations. A much more accurate prognosis can be given for these specific syndromes and this might be more useful than talking about the age, particular seizure type and so forth.

Chadwick: I quite agree. The problem is that we have not yet got a generally agreed international classification of epilepsies, as opposed to seizures. However, these epilepsy syndromes are definable in terms of seizure characteristics, EEG, and age of onset, and we will be interpreting the information we are collecting in this way.

McWilliam: If you disregarded benign cases, you would probably find that the partial seizures have a bad prognosis.

Chadwick: Absolutely, but there are still great disagreements over well-defined epileptic syndromes. For instance, the benign myoclonic epilepsy of adolescence is said by many neurologists to have very high relapse rates, as much as 90%, while others say only 10% will relapse.

Dr S. J. Wallace (Cardiff) Chairman: Considering the pharmacokinetics of phenytoin do you think it should be withdrawn gradually?

Chadwick: Both phenobarbitone and phenytoin have very long half-lives, but many people feel that phenobarbitone withdrawal particularly might cause withdrawal seizures. On the whole I would be cautious about withdrawal, because I don't see many tangible benefits from coming off drugs in one month, as opposed to six months.

Epilepsy in Young People
Edited by E. Ross, D. Chadwick and R. Crawford

8

Cognitive function and epilepsy

JULIE BULLEN
King's College Hospital, London

SUMMARY

The literature suggests that a small subgroup of people with epilepsy show intellectual impairment and/or deterioration. The causes of such effects are not yet clear, although severe fits, which cause neurological damage, and age of the patient at onset of the disease seem important. Severity of the seizure disorder and seizure type may also be of significance but less consistently. There is also evidence that the treatment of epilepsy may contribute to intellectual impairment. Polytherapy and toxicity of certain drugs are implicated. Short-term monotherapy seems to have little impact on specific cognitive functions.

INTRODUCTION

Both epilepsy and its treatment appear to be associated with adverse effects on cognitive functioning. Cognitive functioning is a term used to describe the individual's capacity to analyse and utilize incoming information to coordinate behaviour. It constitutes such specific functions as perception, attention and memory, and complex skills such as reading.

Two main approaches towards the assessment of cognitive functioning have been adopted in studies of epilepsy: *global measures*, such as IQ, and *specific measures* of particular functions or combinations of functions.

INTELLECTUAL ABILITY IN EPILEPSY

Three main questions have been addressed:

1. Are people with epilepsy intellectually impaired relative to those without epilepsy?

2. Do the intellectual functions of people with epilepsy deteriorate over a specified period of follow-up?
3. What factors are related to intellectual impairment and/or deterioration?

Intellectual impairment

Farwell *et al.* (1985) found an average IQ of 93 in a group of 118 people with epilepsy from two tertiary referral centres. This was significantly lower than in a control group matched by age. In contrast, Bourgeois *et al.* (1983) found that a group of untreated people newly diagnosed as having epilepsy had an average IQ of 100 which did not differ significantly from non-affected sibling controls.

Possible explanations for this discrepancy are suggested by Ellenberg *et al.* (1986). Compared with the rest of their sample, collected as part of the Neurological and Communicative Disorder Perinatal Project (NCPP), those with epilepsy emerged as significantly impaired. When controls matched by social class, race and gender were used, however, those with epilepsy were not significantly different. Similarly we found in the King's College Hospital study that the mean IQ in untreated, newly diagnosed patients with epilepsy was below average but the sample was weighted towards the lower social classes. Inconsistencies in the literature may also relate to the extent to which neurological impairment is present in the sample (see below).

Overall, the evidence suggests that when social variables are controlled the majority with epilepsy are not impaired intellectually. Possible explanations for impairment in a subgroup are explored later.

Intellectual deterioration

A number of longitudinal studies of outpatient samples have recently been published. Bourgeois *et al.* (1983) in a prospective study, with an average follow-up of four years, found no significant fall in intelligence in the sample as a whole, but a group of 11.1% did show deterioration. Similarly, Rodin *et al.* (1986) in a retrospective study covering an average of 9.6 years found a subgroup which deteriorated and a larger group which fluctuated markedly. Ellenberg *et al.* (1986) also noted that the IQ of their group with epilepsy was more variable over a three-year period. In the King's College study we also found no evidence of deterioration in the group as a whole (follow-up ranging from 30 to 170 weeks).

Corbett *et al.* (1985) found a sustained fall in IQ of 15 or more points in 15.7% of a sample in a residential school. These recent findings are consistent with earlier studies reviewed by Corbett and Trimble (1983) who concluded that 'a small minority show a progressive fall in intellectual ability'.

Factors related to impairment and deterioration

Brain damage

In a review of brain damage Rodin (1968) concluded that IQ was lowered in children with organic epilepsy while those with non-organic epilepsy had abilities within the normal range with some over-representation in the lower part of the range. This organic link was confirmed by Rutter *et al.* (1970) in the Isle of Wight study and subsequently by Klove and Mathews (1974).

The importance of organic damage is also confirmed in the recent longitudinal studies. Bourgeois *et al.* (1983) showed that those with symptomatic epilepsy had significantly lower IQs than those with idiopathic epilepsy. Rodin *et al.* found that the relation between remission and deterioration was eliminated when only patients with a normal neurological examination were considered. Ellenberg *et al.* (1986) found that the variability of their group over time could be attributed to those showing neurological abnormalities, and this was also true for the occurrence of mental retardation. These findings are particularly interesting as neurological status was measured before the emergence of epilepsy.

Age at onset

Early studies showed little evidence of an association between age of onset and intellectual impairment (Rodin, 1968). Since that review, however, positive evidence of an association has emerged with some consistency (Klove and Mathews, 1974; Dikmen *et al.*, 1977; O'Leary *et al.*, 1981; Farwell *et al.*, 1985). A significant association between early age of onset and intellectual deterioration has been found in longitudinal studies (Bourgeois *et al.*, 1983; Rodin *et al.*, 1983). Corbett *et al.* (1985) report an early age of onset in their sample of children with complicated epilepsy and high rates of impairment.

Severity of seizure disorder

It has been suggested that seizures themselves could cause deterioration, but the data are equivocal and often confounded (Brown and Reynolds, 1981; Corbett and Trimble, 1983). Recent data are equally unclear. Rodin *et al.* (1986) found that their non-remitted group showed a significantly greater loss in performance IQ, but once neurological damage was controlled this finding disappeared. Bourgeois *et al.* (1983) found that their deteriorated group were more often 'difficult to control', i.e. patients had more than 25 seizures of any type between any two-yearly evaluations. Farwell *et al.* (1985) also found that good seizure control correlated with a higher IQ. Neither study provides information on how this factor might relate to other factors. Corbett *et al.* (1985) found no correlation with seizure frequency. This may be attributable to the relative homogeneity of their group in this respect.

Seizure type

Classical absence seizures were found to be related to average or above-average IQ, whereas atypical absence seizures and minor motor seizures, with and without other seizure types, were associated with significantly lower IQs (Farwell *et al.*, 1985). This is consistent with previous research.

The finding by Lennox and Lennox (1960) that people with mixed seizure types are more impaired than those with single seizure types was confirmed by Bourgeois *et al.* (1983). These patients did not deteriorate, however. The only recent study to investigate EEG data found no correlation between deterioration and overall severity of the EEG abnormality (Corbett *et al.*, 1985).

While these recent studies relate to IQ measures, previous research investigated the effect of seizure type using more specific measures of cognitive function. In general they showed that: psychomotor seizures are associated with memory impairment, left hemisphere foci with learning and verbal deficits, right hemisphere foci with spatial problems, and centrencephalic foci with attentional difficulties (review in Brown and Reynolds, 1981).

Interactions

It is important to understand how these factors interact. Scarpa and Carassini (1982) report the worst brain dysfunction in children who experienced onset of seizures within the first year of life. This begs the question of which comes first, and the intriguing finding that prior neurological status was of importance in intellectual stability is of relevance here (Ellenberg *et al.*, 1986).

Frequent seizures plus early age of onset may constitute a particular risk factor in relation to cognitive functioning. Finally, seizure type and brain damage may interact, since major motor seizures plus identifiable neurological insult are associated with greater impairment than minor seizures with no evidence of neurological insult (Corbett and Trimble, 1983).

Anticonvulsant medication

Impaired intellectual performance has been observed in children on long-term phenytoin (Rosen, 1968; Stores, 1977). Recent data is consistent with this view.

Patients with higher serum levels of phenobarbitone showed a lower performance IQ and there was a similar trend for phenytoin (Rodin *et al.*, 1986). This is consistent with Corbett *et al.* (1985) who found that higher levels of phenytoin and primidone correlated with deterioration in IQ. The correlation with phenytoin remained when lower IQ (<70) and high seizure frequency (>10 per month) were excluded. When lower IQs were excluded a correlation between phenobarbitone and performance IQ deterioration emerged. It should be noted that most of the children in this study were on multiple drugs. Bourgeois *et al.*

(1983) found that there was a higher probability of patients being on more than one anticonvulsant at any one time in the group exhibiting deterioration. Phenobarbitone was particularly implicated, with a higher incidence of drug levels in the toxic range.

Global measures such as IQ are inappropriate for the detection of specific cognitive deficits. Furthermore, most studies measuring specific cognitive functions in epilepsy and its treatment have been in adults. However, the evidence from such studies is fairly consistent with the findings reported on IQ in children. For instance, comparing new referrals treated with only carbamazepine or phenytoin, significant differences in favour of carbamazepine were found on a number of memory tasks (Andrewes *et al.*, 1986). In addition, higher serum levels of carbamazepine were significantly related to lower levels of self-reported anxiety, fatigue and depression. Similarly, Thompson and Trimble (1982) found impairment in some measures of memory, and of mental and motor speed, which correlated with serum levels of phenytoin but not of carbamazepine. Concerning polytherapy, Tomlinson *et al.* (1982) and Thompson and Trimble (1982) have shown improvements in memory, concentration and motor speed following reduction in polytherapy.

Studies employing specific measures in children are rare, but some preliminary data from our present study at King's College Hospital illustrate work of this kind. As part of a larger study investigating the relative efficacy and toxicity of major anticonvulsants we compared a subgroup of children with epilepsy with a group of non-epileptic children performing a series of tests of cognitive functioning. All children were tested on three occasions over a nine-month period. For those with epilepsy the first assessment was a pretreatment baseline measure, after which they were randomly assigned to one of three anticonvulsants (phenytoin, carbamazepine or valproate).

The group with epilepsy was found to be significantly slower on a simple reaction-time task and obtained lower scores on a tracking task. The former results may be attributed to computer experience. The tracking task is sensitive to lapses in concentration which is an interesting finding.

These differences were found before treatment and no increased decrement (or improvement) was observed after the onset of treatment. Little evidence was therefore obtained for a detrimental effect of monotherapy over the first nine months of treatment.

CONCLUSIONS

The most difficult task facing the clinician is to balance those hazards arising from the condition being treated against those arising from the treatment. Information is required on the nature of such hazards and their causes. Although this information is not yet complete for cognitive functioning in epilepsy, some consistent findings are emerging.

It is important that future investigations take account of all the epileptic variables discussed in designing and reporting their research. This would allow greater understanding of the interaction of these factors and allow the studies to be combined more readily to produce an advancing body of knowledge. The results of longer follow-up from longitudinal studies in progress should also prove to be of value.

Although there is evidence that the treatment of epilepsy may contribute to intellectual impairment/deterioration, the effects of particular drugs have rarely been assessed separately in children. In addition, more studies are required which measure specific cognitive functions in children and relate these to serum levels of various anticonvulsants.

REFERENCES

ANDREWES, D. G., BULLEN, J. G., TOMLINSON, L., ELWES, R. D. C. and REYNOLDS, E. H. (1986) A comparative study of the cognitive effects of phenytoin and carbamazepine in new referrals with epilepsy. *Epilepsia*, **27**, 128–134.

BOURGEOIS, B. F. D., PRENSKY, A. L., PALKES, H. S., TALENT, B. K. and BUSCIT, S. G. (1983) Intelligence in epilepsy: a prospective study in children. *Ann. Neurol.*, **14**, 438–444.

BROWN, S. W. and REYNOLDS, E. H. (1981) Cognitive impairment in epileptic patients. In: *Epilepsy and Psychiatry*, E. H. Reynolds and M. R. Trimble (Eds), Churchill Livingstone, Edinburgh, pp. 147–164.

CORBETT, J. A. and TRIMBLE, M. R. (1983) Epilepsy and anticonvulsant medication. In: *Developmental Neuropsychiatry*, M. Rutter (Ed.), Guildford Press, New York, pp. 112–129.

CORBETT, J. A. TRIMBLE, M. R. and NICOL, T. C. (1985) Behavioural and cognitive impairments in children with epilepsy: The long term effects of anticonvulsant therapy. *J. Am. Acad. Child Psychiatry*, **24**, 17–23.

DIKMEN, S., MATHEWS, C. G. and HARLEY, J. P. (1977) Effects of early vs late onset of major motor epilepsy on cognitive-intellectual performance: Further considerations. *Epilepsia*, **18**, 31–35.

ELLENBERG, J. H., HIRTZ, D. G. and NELSON, K. B. (1986) Do seizures in children cause intellectual deterioration? *N. Engl. J. Med.*, **314**, 1085–1088.

FARWELL, J. R., DODRILL, C. B. and BATZEL, L. W. (1985) Neurophysiological abilities of children with epilepsy. *Epilepsia*, **26**, 395–400.

KLOVE, H. and MATHEWS, C. G. (1974) Neurophysiological abilities of patients with epilepsy. In: *Clinical Neuropsychology: Current Status and Applications*, M. Reitan and L. A. Davidson (Eds), Wiley, New York, pp. 237–266.

LENNOX, W. G. and LENNOX, M. A. (1960) *Epilepsy and Related Disorders*, Little, Brown, Boston.

O'LEARY, D. S., SEIDENBERG, M., BERENTS, S. and BOLL, T. J. (1981) Effects of age of onset of tonic-clonic seizures on neurophysiological performance in children. *Epilepsia*, **22**, 197–204.

RODIN, E. (1968) *The Prognosis of Patients with Epilepsy*, Charles C. Thomas, Springfield, Illinois.

RODIN, E., SCHMALTZ, S. and TUITLY, G. (1986) Intellectual functions of patients with childhood-onset epilepsy. *Dev. Med. Child Neurol.*, **28**, 25–33.

ROSEN, J. A. (1968) Dilantin Dementia. *Trans. Am. Neurol. Assoc.*, **93**, 273–277.

RUTTER, M., GRAHAM, P. and YULE, W. (1970) A neuropsychiatric study in childhood. *Clinics in Developmental Medicine*, nos. 35–36, Spastics International Medical Publications/Heinemann Medical, London.

SCARPA, P. and CARASSINI, B. (1982) Partial epilepsy in childhood. Clinical and EEG study of 261 cases. *Epilepsia*, **23**, 333–341.

STORES, G. (1977) Behaviour disturbance and type of epilepsy in children attending ordinary schools. In: *Epilepsy*, Proceedings of the VII International Epilepsy Symposium, J. K. Penry (Ed.), Raven Press, New York, pp. 245–249.

THOMPSON, P. J. and TRIMBLE, M. R. (1982) Anticonvulsant drugs and cognitive functions. *Epilepsia*, **23**, 531–544.

TOMLINSON, L. L., ANDREWES, D. G., MERRIFIELD, E. and REYNOLDS, E. H. (1982) The effects of antiepileptic drugs on cognitive and motor functions. *Br. J. Clin. Prac.*, **18** (suppl.), 177–183.

DISCUSSION

Dr J. Corbett (East Grinstead): I would like to compliment Miss Bullen on her excellent review of this topic. May I elaborate on the reference to our own work? The children attended Lingfield Hospital School, which is a special residential school and further education college for young people with epilepsy, most of whom suffer from long-standing and complicated epilepsy. We have recently repeated the cross-sectional study of young people at Lingfield in order to examine further the mechanisms leading to intellectual deterioration. The preliminary results are described in the book *Paediatric Perspectives on Epilepsy* (Ross and Reynolds, 1985).

The main finding cast some doubt on our earlier estimates of the contribution of phenytoin and folate depletion to intellectual impairment, in much the same way that Lennox downgraded his estimates of anticonvulsant effects over the years. While it is possible that subacute phenytoin encephalopathy does occur, the rate of cognitive deterioration was increased (50% of 16%) in the new cohort screened in 1984 compared with those seen in 1976, while the consumption of phenytoin was much reduced (30% of 68%). This finding is almost certainly influenced by selection factors, but detailed investigation of a subgroup with sequential assessment on the Wechsler Intelligence Scale for Children suggests two main conclusions:

1. The intellectual deterioration seen in children with complicated epilepsy is usually non-progressive. The children show a decline in intellectual functioning followed by arrest, but not the progressive impairment seen in dementia.
2. The intellectual deterioration arises from a variety of mechanisms in children with severe epilepsy and these interact, as Miss Bullen has pointed out.

In any individual case is it often difficult to decide whether intellectual deterioration is a result of brain damage or whether persistent brain dysfunction results in some irreversible impairment in learning. There is little evidence at present to suggest that newer drugs such as carbamazepine or valproate are implicated, but it is too early to have a clear picture and it may take many years to evaluate the long-term effects of anticonvulsants on the developing brain.

Finally, a distinction needs to be made between severe and subtle impairment in learning like those seen in newly treated children with epilepsy attending normal schools. Subtle impairments comprise the majority, and the interaction between drugs and other factors may be very important. The less frequent but more obvious non-progressive deterioration which occurs during early childhood in some children with severe epilepsy may be a very important cause of mental handicap.

Bullen: Thank you for your comments and expansion of what I have said. One of the most consistent findings is fluctuation, with progressive fall, in IQ. Longer follow-up should make the picture clearer.

Dr S. J. Wallace (Cardiff), Chairman: Do you have any information about the permanency of any drug effects and whether withdrawal of drugs after two years produces any improvement?

Bullen: Studies done so far show improvements when anticonvulsants are reduced or withdrawn entirely, which suggests that the effects are not permanent. But this is an area for future research, including psychometric testing.

Dr J. Stephenson (Glasgow): Do you have any information on the long-term prognosis of children who begin with above-average intelligence and develop very severe epilepsy with intellectual deterioration from the onset?

Bullen: A few studies indicate that higher initial IQs may show greater falls, but that may be a statistical anomaly in that there is more room for change. This too is an area of interest, where future research may be directed.

REFERENCE

ROSS E. and REYNOLDS, E. (1985) *Paediatric Perspectives on Epilepsy*, Wiley, Chichester, pp. 86–88.

Epilepsy in Young People
Edited by E. Ross, D. Chadwick and R. Crawford

9

Epilepsy, anticonvulsants and pregnancy

MARTIN J. BRODIE
Clinical Pharmacology Unit, University Department of Medicine, Western Infirmary Glasgow

SUMMARY

Seizure control sometimes deteriorates during pregnancy, and circulating anticonvulsant concentrations may fall. The incidence of congenital malformations (ca. 6% of live births) is two to three times that of the normal population, the most frequent being facial clefts and congenital heart defects. Combinations of anticonvulsant drugs carry a risk of fetal malformation of approximately 10%. Recent evidence indicates an increased risk of major neural tube defects in infants born to mothers receiving sodium valproate. Overall, stillbirth and perinatal mortality rates are above-average, and both mother and child may be prone to bleed, the mother at delivery and the infant during the first day of life. The neonate may also experience CNS depression and anticonvulsant withdrawal symptoms. Breast feeding produces few problems. Ideally, the management of pregnancy in women with epilepsy should begin before conception, the aim being to withdraw anticonvulsant therapy if the patient has been seizure-free for some years, or to establish monotherapy at optimal blood levels. Carbamazepine seems to have the least risk of teratogenesis in patients with generalized or partial epilepsy. Ethosuximide may be preferred for absence seizures. Special measures are necessary during pregnancy, delivery and the puerperium, requiring close collaboration.

INTRODUCTION

The spectre of problems in pregnancy is a major concern for the young woman with epilepsy, her husband and her doctors. Ideally, plans should be laid well before conception, and anticonvulsant medication rationalized while contraception is still being practised. Management of the pregnancy itself will involve close cooperation between the obstetrician, general practitioner and, often, the epilepsy specialist. While each individual case will present its own difficulties, substantial knowledge has accumulated over recent years on the effect of pregnancy on seizure frequency, the disposition of anticonvulsant drugs, the risks and prenatal diagnosis of teratogenesis, and the problems for mother and child at delivery and in the puerperium. Such information now contributes to a more coordinated and informed approach to this difficult area of clinical practice.

OBSTETRIC COMPLICATIONS

The effect of pregnancy on seizure control is unpredictable, both between patients and for different pregnancies in the same patient. If fit frequency does change, it is usually for the worse (Dalessio, 1985). Neither maternal age nor family history nor duration of epilepsy appears to influence prognosis during a subsequent pregnancy (Perucca and Richens, 1983). Although there are substantial variations in the figures quoted, the overall picture suggests that around half of women with epilepsy will have no alteration in seizure frequency during pregnancy; about 40% will have more fits than before, and a small proportion will even improve (Schmidt *et al.*, 1983). There is a general consensus that the more severe the seizure disorder, the more likely the pregnancy-related deterioration (Knight and Rhind, 1975). Increased seizure frequency can be expected in the first trimester, during labour and in the puerperium (Philbert and Dam, 1982). Status epilepticus is not common in pregnant women, occurring in less than 1% of pregnancies.

The incidence of hyperemesis gravidarum, abruptio placentae and pre-eclamptic toxaemia is not increased (Bjerkedal and Egenaes, 1982). However, excessive bleeding at delivery may be a problem. Induction of labour and intervention during delivery are more likely and women with epilepsy appear to have a higher overall risk of complications (Egenaes, 1982). It seems wise, therefore, to recommend that such patients be followed particularly closely during pregnancy and at delivery.

ANTICONVULSANT DISPOSITION

Monitoring of drug therapy has been one of the major advances in the management of epilepsy over the past decade. The changes in drug distribution in pregnancy and the effects on circulating anticonvulsant concentrations have now been well worked out in a number of detailed studies. The clinical decision whether or not to alter dosage in response to these changes is not so clear-cut and depends, in part at least, on the closeness of the relationship between concentration and effect for the individual drug in the particular patient.

The changing physiological status of pregnancy may result in increased volume of distribution, decreased protein binding, and augmented hepatic metabolism and renal excretion of drugs (Krauer, 1985). These factors may all contribute to the tendency of circulating anticonvulsant concentrations to fall as pregnancy progresses. Because of the differences in chemical properties between the major anticonvulsants the effect of pregnancy on the pharmacokinetics of each will be considered separately.

Phenytoin

Two factors are known to contribute particularly to the fall in phenytoin concentration during late pregnancy (Landon and Kirkley, 1979). These are a reduction in protein-binding (Rubprah *et al.*, 1980) and an increase in systemic clearance (Dam *et al.*, 1979), the latter in part a consequence of the former. As phenytoin is bound to serum albumin, a fall in protein levels may be reflected by a disproportionate reduction in total phenytoin concentration (Chen *et al.*, 1982). Free concentration measurement would give a better guide to the true extent of the fall. The decline in serum levels is maximal at the time of delivery and is followed by a return to baseline values about one month postpartum. The decision to increase phenytoin dosage should depend on the extent of the fall in circulating levels and the clinical status of the patient. Upward adjustment of dosage should not be a routine manoeuvre in all patients receiving phenytoin monotherapy. If dosage is increased during gestation, there is a risk of phenytoin toxicity in the puerperium, requiring an appropriate reduction after delivery.

Carbamazepine

Despite evidence that carbamazepine clearance is also increased during pregnancy (Dam *et al.*, 1979), the effect on circulating concentration is less clear-cut, with most studies showing very little change (Kuhnz *et al.*, 1983; Battino *et al.*, 1985). This can possibly be explained by a reduction in autoinduction of metabolism in response to the falling concentrations (Macphee and Brodie, 1985). Fluctuations in the level of the active metabolite, carbamazepine 10,11 epoxide, are greater but no consistent pattern has emerged. Nevertheless, an increase in dosage may be necessary in the individual patient if seizure frequency rises or circulating levels fall.

Sodium valproate

In view of the poor correlation between sodium valproate levels and anticonvulsant efficacy, it is unlikely that any decrease in concentration reported in the few patients studied (Philbert and Dam, 1982) will have important clinical repercussions. The recent concern regarding the teratogenic effects of the drug makes it less likely that it will be used in pregnancy in the future.

Phenobarbitone and primidone

Small falls in phenobarbitone and primidone concentrations have been reported by a number of groups but these are less impressive than with phenytoin (Perucca and Richens, 1983). Similarly, levels of phenobarbitone may decline in patients receiving primidone, for which it is a major metabolite (Nau *et al.*, 1982). These changes may be a consequence of decreased protein binding together with augmentation of metabolism. The limited alterations in the circulating levels of these drugs compared with phenytoin reflect their lower protein binding and, possibly, the availability of a renal route of elimination for phenobarbitone.

TERATOGENESIS

The incidence of congenital malformations in children born to mothers with epilepsy is generally agreed to be two to three times that of the normal population (Kelly, 1984). An overall figure of 6% is usually quoted (Boobis, 1978). There seems little doubt that this increase is partly a consequence of anticonvulsant teratogenesis and partly due to poor seizure control. The most frequently observed abnormalities are cleft lip and palate and congenital heart defects. The incidence of each in women with epilepsy is around 18 per 1000 births, compared to two per 1000 for facial clefts and five per 1000 births for congenital heart disease in the rest of the population (Perucca and Richens, 1983). A combination of anticonvulsant drugs, particularly in excess of two, carries a substantial risk (ca. 10%) of fetal malformations (Nakana *et al.*, 1980). This may be due to a synergistic effect of more severe disease with higher numbers and doses of anticonvulsant drugs. A recent report of increased incidence of neural tube defects in neonates of mothers receiving sodium valproate (Lindhout and Schmidt, 1986) gives cause for concern.

Phenytoin

Phenytoin is the anticonvulsant agent for which the greatest evidence of teratogenicity has accumulated. Up to 30% of exposed fetuses have been reported to show minor craniofacial and digital anomalies of varying degrees (Kelly, 1984). These form part of a disputed 'fetal hydantoin syndrome' (Table 1) which includes broad low nasal bridge, epicanthic folds, hypertelorism, ocular abnormalities, slightly malformed ears, wide mouth with prominent lips, and hypoplasia of the distal phalanges and nails (Anon, 1981). There may also be relative microcephaly and a degree of mental retardation. In about 10% of neonates a sufficient number of these features can be identified to support the existence of a specific syndrome (Hanson *et al.*, 1976). There have also been some recent, if rather rare, worrying reports associating phenytoin with the later development of neuroblastoma (Ehrenbard and Chaganti, 1981).

Table 1. Features of the 'fetal hydantoin syndrome'

Dysmorphic features	Abnormalities of growth
Short nose with depressed bridge	Prenatal and postnatal growth deficiency
Hypertelorism and epicanthic folds	Relative micrencephaly
Ocular abnormalities	Mild mental retardation
Malformed ears	Developmental delay
Wide mouth and prominent lips	
Short neck	
Hypoplasia of distal phalanges and nails	
Cleft lip and palate	

Sodium valproate

The teratogenic potential of sodium valproate has been the subject of much debate despite conclusive evidence of morphological abnormalities in animals (Anon, 1982). Evidence is now accumulating that the drug is responsible for a significant specific increase in serious neural tube defects, particularly spina bifida (Robert and Guibaud, 1982, Bjerkedal *et al.*, 1982; Garden *et al.*, 1985). The figures may be as high as 1–2% of fetuses exposed to the drug in the first trimester of pregnancy (Lindhout and Schmidt, 1986), a risk 10 times that of the background incidence. These findings are particularly important as the abnormalities are severe and, in the main, untreatable, while the drug is particularly effective for the management of centrencephalic epilepsy in young patients. From the limited information available, ethosuximide appears relatively safe in pregnancy, and this drug may be preferred for the treatment of absence seizures in women of childbearing age (Fabro and Brown, 1979).

Phenobarbitone and primidone

The evidence that phenobarbitone and primidone, when given as monotherapy, may be associated with significant teratogenesis is surprisingly slight despite many years of clinical use. An increased incidence of cleft palate and cardiac malformations has been reported (Annegers *et al.*, 1974), but most abnormalities occur when these drugs are used in combination with phenytoin (Fedrick, 1973). Since primidone is partly metabolized to phenobarbitone, this drug might be expected to have comparable or greater teratogenic potential than its metabolite and a number of malformations have, indeed, been described (Rudd and Freedom, 1979). A Finnish study recently reported that the mean head circumference of babies born to mothers on phenobarbitone-containing anticonvulsant combinations was 6mm less than that of controls (Hiilesmaa *et al.*, 1981). The clinical relevance of this observation is unknown. However, Gold *et al.* (1978) reported an increased risk of brain tumours in children of mothers who received barbiturates during pregnancy.

Carbamazepine

Despite 20 years of clinical use, carbamazepine monotherapy has a relatively 'clean' profile in pregnancy. The drug has been reported to reduce the mean head circumference of exposed infants by 7mm (Hiilesmaa *et al.*, 1981). Most of the individual values remained within the normal range and no evidence was presented to support an effect on cerebral function. As with all other anticonvulsants, combinations which include carbamazepine may produce an increased risk of fetal malformation, which could be a consequence of increased production of the active metabolite, carbamazepine 10,11 epoxide (Lindhout *et al.*, 1984).

NEONATAL PROBLEMS

The offspring of mothers with epilepsy have been reported to have higher stillbirth (Fedrick, 1973) and perinatal mortality (Bjerkedal and Bahna, 1978) rates than those in the general population. This may be, in part, a consequence of anticonvulsant therapy (Monson *et al.*, 1973). Babies born to women with treated epilepsy are lighter than controls (Bjerkedal, 1982) and may have smaller heads (Perucca and Richens, 1983). Frank microcephaly is rare.

All anticonvulsant drugs cross the placenta and, theoretically, may produce central nervous system depression in the neonate (Nau *et al.*, 1982). This appears particularly likely with high-dose diazepam, given to the mother at the time of delivery, which may result in prolonged neonatal sedation with a low Apgar score (Cree *et al.*, 1973). Lower doses of benzodiazepines taken chronically during pregnancy may also sedate the newborn but to a lesser degree (Gillberg, 1977). Phenobarbitone, primidone and phenytoin may produce some CNS depression but, as a rule, low Apgar scores do not occur more frequently in babies of epileptic mothers than in controls. The most commonly encountered symptoms in such infants are vomiting and sucking difficulties. These may be partly explained by a mild abstinence syndrome, particularly if the infant is exposed *in utero* to phenobarbitone or primidone (Desmond *et al.*, 1972). Other features may include overactivity, restlessness, poor sleeping, hyperreflexia and diarrhoea. Seizures rarely occur. These symptoms may take a month or two to settle (Perucca and Richens, 1983). Paradoxical hyperactivity may be due to withdrawal of transplacental benzodiazepines (Rementeria and Bhatt, 1977). The possibility of a withdrawal syndrome has also been mooted with phenytoin (Hill *et al.*, 1974), but not following treatment with carbamazepine, ethosuximide or sodium valproate.

A bleeding tendency may develop during the first day of life in neonates exposed to phenytoin, phenobarbitone or primidone. This is a consequence of decreased levels of vitamin-K-dependent clotting factors and may be life-threatening (Bleyer and Skinner, 1976). Haemorrhagic screening is normal in the mother but not in the infant, in whom prothrombin and partial thromboplastin times may be prolonged. Bleeding can be prevented by injections of phytomenadione (vitamin K_1) given to the mother before delivery and to the neonate shortly after birth. If it becomes apparent, fresh-frozen plasma or commercially prepared concentrates of factors II, VII, IX and X can be used. The bleeding may be a consequence of enzyme induction in the fetus, particularly if anticonvulsant combinations are employed. It may also contribute toward neonatal deficiency of folic acid (Boobis, 1978) and vitamin D (Friis and Sandemann, 1977). Finally, transient gingival hyperplasia has been seen in a few infants exposed to phenytoin *in utero* (Hill *et al.*, 1974).

BREAST FEEDING

All antiepileptic drugs are excreted in breast milk (Nau et al., 1982). However, as all the major anticonvulsants are highly protein-bound, acidic or neutral compounds, milk concentrations can be expected to be lower than those found in maternal serum (Brodie, 1986). As a general rule, breast feeding should be encouraged. No problems have been encountered with carbamazepine, sodium valproate, phenytoin or ethosuximide. Undue neonatal sedation may occasionally be produced if the lactating mother is receiving high doses of phenobarbitone, primidone or, possibly, one of the newer benzodiazepines (Perucca and Richens, 1983). Should this occur, breast feeding is best discontinued.

MANAGEMENT

The management of pregnancy in a woman with epilepsy should ideally begin before conception. The first consideration must be whether anticonvulsant medication is still required. If the patient has been seizure-free for a number of years and does not have evidence of an anatomical cerebral lesion, she should be offered withdrawal of therapy. If continued treatment is essential, monotherapy should be employed whenever possible. The increased risk of oral cleft defects and congenital heart disease is more likely with phenytoin and, possibly, phenobarbitone and primidone, and the risk of neural tube defects with sodium valproate. Carbamazepine monotherapy seems to offer the least likelihood of teratogenesis and is suitable for patients with generalized tonic-clonic or partial epilepsy. Ethosuximide may be a safer choice than sodium valproate for absence seizures. Prior to conception, anticonvulsant concentrations should be brought within the target range for each drug as circulating levels tend to fall during pregnancy. If a patient receiving sodium valproate conceives, prenatal screening for spina bifida, using ultrasound together with amniocentesis and alpha-fetoprotein measurement, will detect more than

Table 2. Summary of management

Pre-conception
Withdraw anticonvulsants if possible
Stabilize on appropriate monotherapy
Optimize circulating anticonvulsant concentrations
Pregnancy
Restrict weight gain and fluid retention
Ensure iron and folate supplementation
Monitor anticonvulsant levels
Adjust dosage upwards if necessary
Delivery
Admit to hospital
Monitor fetus during and immediately after delivery
Administer vitamin K_1
Puerperium
Observe neonate carefully for CNS withdrawal symptoms
Review anticonvulsant concentrations and dosage
Encourage breast feeding

95% of abnormal infants in the first 20 weeks of gestation (Weinbaum *et al.*, 1986). If such a lesion is discovered, therapeutic abortion can be considered.

Weight gain should be monitored and kept to a minimum during pregnancy, fluid retention treated, and iron and low-dose folic acid prescribed (Anon, 1980). The patient should be reviewed regularly by her general practitioner, obstetrician and hospital clinic, with close monitoring of anticonvulsant concentrations. If seizure frequency increases or drug levels fall appreciably, dosage may need to be increased for the duration of the pregnancy. Delivery should be in hospital where fetal monitoring can be undertaken. If phenytoin, phenobarbitone, primidone or, theoretically, carbamazepine therapy has been employed, parenteral vitamin K_1 treatment is necessary for the mother before delivery and for the infant immediately post-partum, to reduce the risk of haemorrhage.

Careful observation of the newborn infant for apnoeic episodes and poor sucking is advisable, particularly if the mother is receiving phenobarbitone, primidone or one of the benzodiazepines. The paediatrician should be alert to any symptoms of an anticonvulsant abstinence syndrome in the first month of life. Continued measurement of anticonvulsant levels in the puerperium is essential if dosage has been increased during pregnancy. Breast feeding should be encouraged and the parents invited to report any evidence of undue sedation in the baby.

Throughout the whole pre-pregnancy period, gestation and puerperium, full and careful discussion of the risks and potential problems should be undertaken with the patient and her husband. They should be invited to take part in the decision-making at each stage. Encouragement is necessary at all times, and a positive approach should be adopted, stressing the likely satisfactory outcome.

Although the patient should be advised that she has a greater than 90% chance of having a normal baby, it is essential that she be made aware that the risk of congenital malformation is two to three times more than in an epilepsy-free patient. With greater understanding of pregnancy-associated problems and the move to monotherapy, future studies may well show an improved prognosis for the epileptic mother and her child.

ACKNOWLEDGEMENT

I would like to thank Anne Somers for expert secretarial assistance.

REFERENCES

ANNEGERS, J. F., ELVEBACK, L. R., HAUSER, W. A. and KURLAND, L. T. (1974) Do anticonvulsants have a teratogenic effect? *Arch. Neurol.*, **31**, 364–373.

ANON (1980) Epilepsy and pregnancy. *Br. Med. J.*, **281**, 1087–1088.

ANON (1981) Teratogenic risk of antiepileptic drugs. *Br. Med. J.*, **283**, 515–516.

ANON (1982) Valproate and malformations. *Lancet*, **ii**, 1313–1314.

BATTINO, D., BINELLI, S., BOSSI, L., CANGER, R., CROCI, D., CUSI, C., DE GIAMBATTISTA, M. and AVANZINI, G. (1985) Plasma concentrations of carbamazepine and carbamazepine 10,11 epoxide during pregnancy and after delivery. *Clin. Pharmacokinet.*, **10**, 279–284.

BJERKEDAL, T. (1982) Outcome of pregnancy in women with epilepsy: Norway 1967–78. 3. Gestational age, birth weight and survival of the newborn. In: *Epilepsy, Pregnancy and the Child*, D. Janz *et al.* (Eds), Raven Press, New York, pp. 175–178.

BJERKEDAL, T. and BAHNA, L. (1978) The course and outcome of pregnancy in women with epilepsy. *Acta Obstet. Gynecol. Scand.*, **52**, 245–248.

BJERKEDAL, T. and EGENAES, J. (1982) Outcome of pregnancy in women with epilepsy: Norway 1967–78. 1. Description of material. In: *Epilepsy, Pregnancy and the Child*, D. Janz *et al.* (Eds), Raven Press, New York, pp. 75–80.

BJERKEDAL, T., CZEIZEL, A., GOUJARD, J., KALLEN, B., MASTROIACOVA, P., NEVIN, N., OAKLEY, G. and ROBERT, E. (1982) Valproic acid and spina bifida. *Lancet*, **ii**, 1096.

BLEYER, W. A. and SKINNER, A. L. (1976) Fatal neonatal haemorrhage after maternal anticonvulsant therapy. *JAMA*, **235**, 626–627.

BOOBIS, S. (1978) The teratogenicity of antiepileptic drugs. *Pharmacol. Ther.*, **2**, 269–283.

BRODIE, M. J. (1986) Drugs and breast feeding. *Practitioner*, **230**, 483–485.

CHEN, S. S., PERUCCA, E., LEE, J.-N. and RICHENS, A. (1982) Serum protein binding and free concentration of phenytoin and phenobarbitone in pregnancy. *Br. J. Clin. Pharmacol.*, **13**, 547–552.

CREE, J. E., MEYER, J. and HAILEY, D. M. (1973) Diazepam in labour: its metabolism and effect on the clinical condition and teratogenesis in the newborn. *Br. Med. J.*, **4**, 251–255.

DALESSIO, D. J. (1985) Seizure disorders in pregnancy. *N. Engl. J. Med.*, **312**, 559–563.

DAM, M., CHRISTIANSEN, J., MUNCK, O. and MYGIND, K. I. (1979) Antiepileptic drugs: Metabolism and pregnancy. *Clin. Pharmacokinet.*, **4**, 53–62.

DESMOND, M. M., SCHWANECHE, R. P., WILSON, G. S., YASUNAGA, S. and BURGDORFF, I. (1972) Maternal barbiturate utilisation and neonatal withdrawal symptomatology. *J. Pediatr.*, **80**, 190–197.

EGENAES, J. (1982) Outcome of pregnancy in women with epilepsy: Norway 1967–78. 2. Complications during pregnancy and delivery. In: *Epilepsy, Pregnancy and the Child*, D. Janz *et al.* (Eds), Raven Press, New York, pp. 81–85.

EHRENBARD, L. T. and CHAGANTI, R. S. K. (1981) Cancer in the fetal hydantoin syndrome. *Lancet*, **ii**, 97.

FABRO, S. and BROWN, N. A. (1979) Teratogenic potential of anticonvulsants. *N. Engl. J. Med.*, **300**, 1280–1281.

FEDRICK, J. (1973) Epilepsy and pregnancy: a report from the Oxford Record Linkage Survey. *Br. Med. J.*, **2**, 442.

FRIIS, B. and SANDEMANN, H. (1977) Neonatal hypocalcaemia after intra-uterine exposure to anticonvulsant drugs. *Arch. Dis. Child.*, **52**, 239–247.

GARDEN, A. S., BENZIE, R. J., HUTTON, E. M. and GARE, D. J. (1985) Valproic acid therapy and neural tube defects. *Can. Med. Assoc. J.*, **132**, 933–934.

GILLBERG, C. (1977) Floppy infant syndrome and maternal diazepam. *Lancet*, **ii**, 244.

GOLD, E., GORDIS, L., TONASCIA, J. and SZKLO, M. (1978) Increased risk of brain tumours in children exposed to barbiturates. *J. Natl. Cancer Inst.*, **61**, 1031–1034.

HANSON, J. W., MYRIANTHOPOULOS, N. C., HARVEY, M. A. S. and SMITH, D. W. (1976) Risks to the offspring of women treated with hydantoin anticonvulsants, with emphasis on the fetal hydantoin syndrome. *J. Pediatr.*, **89**, 662–668.

HIILESMAA, V. K., TERAMO, K., GANSTROM, M. L. and BRADY, A. H. (1981) Fetal head growth retardation associated with maternal antiepileptic drugs. *Lancet*, **ii**, 165–167.

HILL, R. M., VERNIAUD, W. M., HORNING, M. E., MCCULLEY, L. B. and MORGAN, L. F. (1974) Infants exposed *in utero* to antiepileptic drugs. A prospective study. *Am. J. Dis. Child.*, **127**, 645–653.

KELLY, T. D. (1984) Teratogenicity of anticonvulsant drugs. 1. Review of the literature. *Am. J. Med. Genet.*, **19**, 413–434.

KNIGHT, A. H. and RHIND, E. G. (1975) Epilepsy and pregnancy: a study of 153 pregnancies in 59 patients. *Epilepsia*, **16**, 99–110.

KRAUER, B. (1985) Pharmacotherapy during pregnancy: emphasis on pharmacokinetics. In: *Drug Therapy During Pregnancy*, T. K. A. B. Eskes and M. Finster (Eds), Butterworth, London, pp. 9–31.

KUHNZ, W., JAGER-ROMAN, E., RATING, D., DEICHI, A., KUNZE, J., HELGE, H. and NAU, H. (1983) Carbamazepine and carbamazepine 10,11 epoxide during pregnancy and postnatal period in epileptic mothers and their nursed infants: pharmacokinetics and clinical effects. *Pediatr. Pharmacol.*, **3**, 199–208.

LANDON, M. J. and KIRKLEY, M. (1979) Metabolism of diphenyl-hydantoin (phenytoin) during pregnancy. *Br. J. obstet. Gynaecol.*, **86**, 125–132.

LINDHOUT, D. and SCHMIDT, D. (1986) *In-utero* exposure to valproate and neural tube defects. *Lancet*, **i**, 1392–1393.

LINDHOUT, D., HOPPENER, R. J. E. A. and MEINARDI, H. (1984) Teratogenicity of antiepileptic drug combinations with special emphasis on epoxidation (of carbamazepine). *Epilepsia*, **25**, 77–83.

MACPHEE, G. J. A. and BRODIE, M. J. (1985) Carbamazepine substitution in severe partial epilepsy: implication of autoinduction of metabolism. *Postgrad. Med. J.*, **61**, 779–783.

MONSON, R. R., ROSENBERG, L., HARTZ, S. C., SHAPIRO, O. P. and SLOAN, D. (1973) Diphenylhydantoin and selected congenital malformations. *N. Engl. J. Med.*, **289**, 1049–1052.

NAKANA, Y., OKUMA, T., TAKAHASHI, R., SATO, Y., WADA, T., SATO, T., FUKUSHIMA, Y., KUMASHIRO, H., ONO, T., TAKAHASHI, T., AOKI, Y., KAZAMATSURI, H.,

INAMI, M., KOMAI, S., SEINO, M., MIYAKOSHI, M., TANIMURA, T., HAZAMI, H., KAWAHARA, R., OTSUKI, S., HOSOKAWA, K., INANAGA, K., NAKAZAWA, Y. and YAMAMOTO, K. (1980) Multi-institutional study on the teratogenicity and fetal toxicity of antiepileptic drugs: a report of a collaborative study group in Japan. *Epilepsia*, **21**, 663–680.

NAU, H., KUHNZ, W., EGGER, H.-J., RATING, D. and HELGE, H. (1982) Anticonvulsants during pregnancy and lactation: transplacental, maternal and neonatal pharmacokinetics. *Clin. Pharmacokinet.*, **7**, 508–543.

PERUCCA, E. and RICHENS, A. (1983) Antiepileptic drugs, pregnancy and the newborn. In: *Clinical Pharmacology in Obstetrics*, P. J. Lewis (Ed.), Wright PSG, Bristol, pp. 264–288.

PHILBERT, A. and DAM, M. (1982) The epileptic mother and her child. *Epilepsia*, **23**, 85–99.

REMENTERIA, J. C. and BHATT, K. (1977) Withdrawal symptoms in neonates from intrauterine exposure to diazepam. *J. Pediatr.*, **90**, 123–126.

ROBERT, E. and GUIBAUD, P. (1982) Maternal valproic acid and congenital neural tube defects. *Lancet*, **ii**, 937.

RUBPRAH, M., PERUCCA, E. and RICHENS, A. (1980) Decreased serum protein binding of phenytoin in late pregnancy. *Lancet*, **ii**, 316–317.

RUDD, N. L. and FREEDOM, R. M. (1979) A possible primidone embryopathy. *J. Pediatr.*, **94**, 835–837.

SCMIDT, D., CANGER, R., AVANZINI, G., BATTINO, D., CUSI, C., BECK-MANNAGETTA, G., KOCH, S., RATING, D. and JANZ, D. (1983) Changes of seizure frequency in pregnant epileptic women. *J. Neurol. Neurosurg. Psychiatry*, **46**, 751–755.

WEINBAUM, P. J., CASSIDY, S. B., VINTZILEOS, A. M., CAMBELL, W. A., CIARLELGLIO, L. and NOCHIMSON, D. J. (1986) Prenatal detection of a neural tube defect after fetal exposure to valproic acid. *Obstet. Gynecol.*, **67**, 31–33S.

DISCUSSION

Dr J. S. Duncan (Chalfont Centre): Is there any evidence that antiepileptic drugs taken by a child's father may be teratogenic?

Brodie: I'm not aware of any. If this produced a problem, it would probably be abortion, and there is said to be an increased incidence of this. Teratogenesis seems less likely.

Dr Y. F. Ransley (Epsom): Do you know whether any of the patients who produced spina bifida babies in Smithells' study (1976; also Wald and Cuckle, 1984) were on antiepileptic drugs? And would vitamin B complex in the pregnancy be effective in preventing spina bifida?

Brodie: As far as I am aware, there were no such patients. Whether vitamin supplements would have a prophylactic effect in valproate-associated spina bifida is not known. The mechanism by which valproate appears to cause this problem has yet to be elucidated, and prospective studies present major problems. It may be more practicable to take patients off valproate if conception is likely or possibly avoid the drug, if possible, for treatment in young women if the association with spina bifida is confirmed.

Dr D. W. Chadwick (Liverpool): This is a very important question because valproate is a particularly effective drug against many of the epilepsies that occur in young women. Screening any pregnancies that occur in patients on valproate is clearly vital, and we should also bear in mind that there may be an increased incidence of neural-tube defects from pregnancies where the mother was taking other drugs. I am particularly concerned because I recently had a pregnant patient on valproate who underwent ultrasound examination but not amniocentesis (for domestic, not medical, reasons) and unfortunately had a stillbirth with a gross neural-tube defect. How conclusively can neural-tube defects be identified or excluded in early pregnancy?

Brodie: In about 90–95% of cases, according to the literature (Weinbaum *et al.*, 1986). But serious problems still arise in those patients for whom abortion is not a possibility.

REFERENCE

SMITHELLS, R. W. *et al.* (1976) Vitamin deficiency and neural tube defects. *Arch. Dis. Child.*, **51**, 944–50.

WALD, N. J. and CUCKLE, H. S. (1984) Open neural tube defects. In: Antenatal and neonatal screening, N. J. Wald (Ed.), Oxford University Press, pp. 25–73.

WEINBAUM, P. J., CASSIDY, S. B., VINTZILEOS, A. M. CAMPBELL, W. A., CIARLELGLIO, L. and NOCHIMSON, D. J. (1986) Prenatal detection of a neural tube defect after fetal exposure to valproic acid. *Obstet. Gynecol.*, **67**, 31–33S.

Epilepsy in Young People
Edited by E. Ross, D. Chadwick and R. Crawford

10

New anticonvulsant drugs and their development

PAMELA M. CRAWFORD
North Manchester General Hospital

SUMMARY

There is a need for new anticonvulsant drugs with greater efficacy and less toxicity, since 10% of patients continue to have recurrent seizures despite optimal conventional therapy. A greater understanding of the pathophysiological events underlying seizure activity and the establishment of a major drug development programme in the USA have led to the development of more than ten new putative antiepileptic agents in the last five years. These new compounds include the first drugs to be developed on a rational basis, progabide and vigabatrin, both of which have actions on the GABAergic inhibitory system.

INTRODUCTION

Recent studies have emphasized the good prognosis of patients with newly diagnosed epilepsy. However, about 10% of patients present management problems and continue to have seizures despite anticonvulsant therapy. These patients gravitate towards hospital clinics and polypharmacy. The problems they suffer demonstrate the need for new anticonvulsant drugs.

Important questions need to be answered in the clinical evaluation of any new putative anticonvulsant drug:

1. Is the drug effective and against which seizure type?
2. What are its side-effects?
3. How do its efficacy and toxicity compare with current anticonvulsant drugs?

DEVELOPMENT STRATEGIES

In the past, newly synthesized compounds were screened for antiseizure activity against a wide range of animal seizure models. However, in more recent years, advances in our understanding of the neurochemical basis of epilepsy have led to a more rational development of new anticonvulsant drugs. Attention has been focused on gamma aminobutyric acid (GABA), the major inhibitory neurotransmitter in the mammalian CNS (Fig. 1). Any drug which decreases the synthesis of GABA, or blocks its binding to its receptor site or chloride ion channel, leads to convulsions. Conversely any agent which enhances GABAergic action is likely to be anticonvulsant in a wide range of animal models. The GABAergic system is involved in many of the anticonvulsant actions of anticonvulsant drugs now in use, although its role in the aetiology of human epilepsy, apart from vitamin B_6 deficiency, is unclear (Spero, 1982).

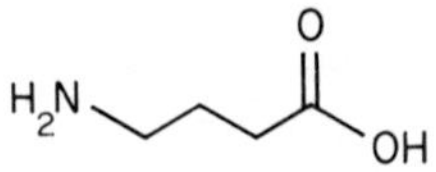

Fig. 1 Chemical structure of GABA

NEW GABA-RELATED DRUGS

Progabide

Progabide (Fig. 2) is a specific GABA agonist which readily crosses the blood-brain barrier. Open studies in man appeared to show a considerable beneficial effect, though more recent studies have failed to confirm this initial optimism (Table 1). Three major studies have been unable to differentiate the anticonvulsant effects of progabide from placebo (Dam *et al.*, 1983; Schmidt and Utech, 1985; Crawford and Chadwick, 1986).

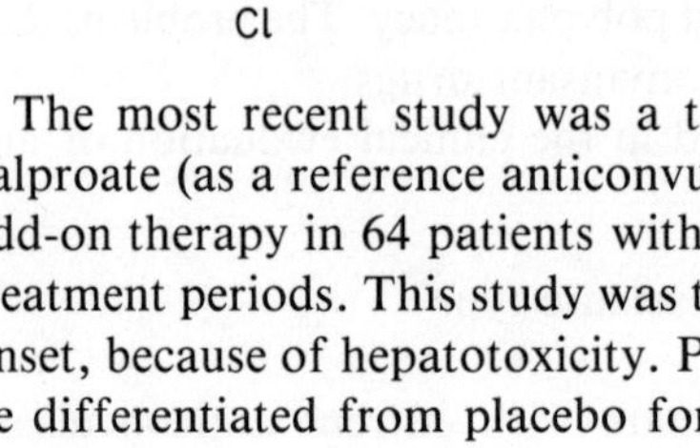

Fig. 2. Chemical structure of progabide

The most recent study was a three-way crossover of progabide, sodium valproate (as a reference anticonvulsant with proven efficacy) and placebo as add-on therapy in 64 patients with refractory epilepsy, using three six-month treatment periods. This study was terminated prematurely, 18 months after its onset, because of hepatotoxicity. Progabide's anticonvulsant action could not be differentiated from placebo for any seizure type ($p<0.4$). Valproate was significantly superior to placebo ($p<0.0001$) and to progabide ($p<0.009$),

Table 1. Double-blind studies with progabide

Author	*n*	Length of study	Improvement > 50%
Van Parys *et al.* (1985)	20	2×4 weeks	25% ns
Dam *et al.* (1983)	20	2×3 months	5% $p<0.1$
Schmidt and Utech (1985)	19	2×3 months	5% ns
Martinez-Lage *et al.* (1984)	20	2×6 weeks	47% $p<0.01$ (7/15)
Loiseau *et al.* (1983)	24	2×6 weeks	40% $p<0.05$* (8/20)
Weber *et al.* (1985)	20	2×6 weeks	40% $p<0.05$* (8/18)
Kulakowski *et al.* (1985)	18	2×4 weeks	50% $p<0.02$* (9/18)
Crawford and Chadwick (1986)	64	3×6 months	24% $p<0.4$†

Improvement >50% = Reduction in seizures compared with seizure frequencies on placebo
*Studies which include children
†Studies with a third treatment phase of sodium valproate, used as a reference anticonvulsant

demonstrating that the patients studied were capable of improvement with the addition of a new anticonvulsant agent (Crawford and Chadwick, 1986). Palminteri *et al.* (1985) have reported that 8.4% of patients treated with progabide develop elevated transaminases with a cumulative frequency of 14% at one year (26% in elderly patients), and about 0.5% of patients develop clinical hepatitis. This appears to limit the use of progabide, especially when no preferential antiepileptic properties compared to valproate can be demonstrated.

Vigabatrin (γ-vinyl GABA)

Vigabatrin (Fig. 3) is a selective irreversible inhibitor of GABA-transaminase, one of the major degradative enzymes of GABA. Vigabatrin enhances GABAergic inhibitory actions by blocking further metabolism of GABA in both glia and neurones, leading to a sustained dose-dependent increase in cerebral GABA concentrations (Jung *et al.*, 1977; Chapman *et al.*, 1982).

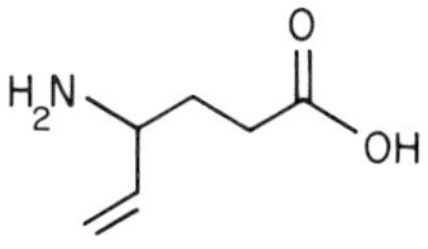

Fig 3. Chemical structure of γ-vinyl GABA

Vigabatrin is an effective anticonvulsant in animal models. However, toxicity studies in rats and dogs led to delay in granting a full clinical trial certificate due to the development of intramyelinic oedema and vacuolation. More recently monkeys treated for 16 months failed to show adverse clinical effects, and postmortem demonstrated little, if any, intramyelinic oedema (Gibson, 1985); further clinical studies may therefore be performed in the UK.

Studies with vigabatrin in humans suggest that it is an effective anticonvulsant. In two double-blind placebo-controlled studies, nine out of 18 and 14 out of

21 patients had a greater than 50% reduction in seizures (Rimmer and Richens, 1984; Gram *et al.*, 1985). No serious side-effects in man have been reported. Vigabatrin therefore appears to be a useful and effective anticonvulsant in those patients with partial epilepsies who are often refractory to conventional therapy.

Gabapentin

Gabapentin (Fig. 4) was designed as a GABA analogue, but animal studies have failed to define any specific pharmacological actions of the drug on GABAergic function. It is, however, active against seizures in animal models, particularly those related to GABAergic dysfunction.

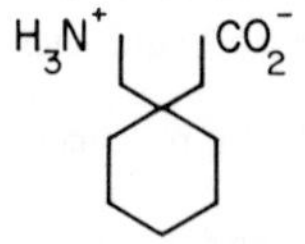

Fig. 4 Chemical structure of gabapentin

An open study in Germany using gabapentin as add-on therapy in about 60 therapy-resistant patients is still under way, but early reports indicate that about 30% of patients have had a greater than 50% reduction in seizures. A dose-finding study comparing three different doses of gabapentin (300 mg, 600 mg and 900 mg) in a double-blind trial design (three periods of two months each, after a two-month baseline period), resulted in 45% of patients with refractory epilepsy having a greater than 50% reduction in seizures ($p<0.0001$) (Crawford *et al.*, 1987). The 900 mg/day dose was significantly more effective than either of the other two. No serious side-effects were reported and 15 patients have continued on long-term gabapentin. Follow-up is now available for one year, and tolerance does not appear to have developed.

Taurine and related compounds

No adequate placebo-controlled clinical trial with taurine has been reported. The proportion of patients responding in open studies has varied from zero to 90%, and tolerance appears to develop (Chadwick and Crawford, 1986). A recent study using taltrimide, a lipophilic derivative of taurine, showed a significant deterioration in seizure control in 16 out of 20 institutionalized patients ($p<0.002$) (Koivisto *et al.*, 1986). Therefore taurine and its analogues are of uncertain value in human epilepsy, despite anticonvulsant action in animal models.

NEW ANTICONVULSANTS DEVELOPED FROM SCREENING PROGRAMMES

Zonisamide

Zonisamide is chemically distinct from currently used anticonvulsants. In animal models it has a similar anticonvulsant profile to phenytoin and carbamazepine but, like phenytoin, it possesses non-linear pharmacokinetics and a narrow therapeutic range (20–30 μg/ml). Side-effects (mental slowing, slowing of speech and dysarthria) develop at concentrations of about 30 μg/ml.

An open pilot study using zonisamide as add-on therapy in 11 patients with refractory partial seizures resulted in nine having a greater than 40% reduction in partial seizures, although this was associated in two patients with an increase in tonic-clonic seizures. Side-effects were frequent and included impairment of cognitive function in various psychological tests (Sachellares *et al.*, 1985).

Preliminary results from two open studies in Japan have been reported. One, an open add-on study in 30 drug-resistant patients, showed that 12 had a significant reduction in seizure frequency; eight complained of mental and physical slowing (Yagi *et al.*, 1985). The second study was an open multicentre study of zonisamide as add-on therapy in 131 patients, 49% of whom had a global improvement in seizure frequency (Seino, 1985).

In another study (Wilensky *et al.*, 1985), eight patients with refractory partial seizures (one or more a week) were maintained for eight weeks on baseline phenytoin monotherapy. They were then randomly allocated to two three-month periods of monotherapy with carbamazepine or zonisamide. Only four patients completed the study; overall, two out of six had a greater than 50% reduction of seizures on carbamazepine, compared to three out of eight on zonisamide. Another three of these eight patients had a more than 100% deterioration in seizure frequency on zonisamide. Major side-effects were reported in all patients receiving zonisamide, including speech problems (six patients) and mental slowing (five patients). There was a significant reduction in verbal and full scale IQ scores in patients on zonisamide, compared with carbamazepine, suggesting that zonisamide therapy is associated with a decrease in mental skills. However, serum concentrations were at the upper limit or above the therapeutic range.

Therefore, although zonisamide appears to have anticonvulsant actions, its non-linear pharmacokinetics, narrow therapeutic range and effects on cognitive function may limit its use.

Flunarizine

Flunarizine is a long-acting difluoro-derivative of cinnarizine. It is a calcium antagonist and probably acts as an anticonvulsant by limiting the spread of seizure activity. In an initial open study, six out of ten patients showed a decrease in seizure frequency. In a double-blind crossover study of two three-month periods of therapy with 10 mg/day flunarizine vs placebo as add-on therapy seven out of 30 patients had a greater than 50% reduction in seizures (Binnie *et al.*, 1985). Serum concentrations were low, so a further dose-finding study was undertaken (Overweg *et al.*, 1984). Increasing doses of 10, 15, 20 and 25 mg of flunarizine were added at three-monthly intervals, relative to the control group, until side-effects occurred or there was a significant reduction in seizure frequency. Fifty-two patients were recruited, 47 of whom completed the study. Sixteen patients had a greater than 50% reduction in seizures and three became seizure-free on 15–20 mg/day of flunarizine. Although no major side-effects were reported in these studies, a recent report has suggested that flunarizine therapy can produce extrapyramidal syndromes similar to the neuroleptics (Chousa *et al.*, 1986).

Lamotrigine (BW 430-C)

Lamotrigine was designed as a folate antagonist and is a novel anticonvulsant with a phenytoin-like profile in animal tests, possibly acting on sodium channels to stabilize neuronal membranes and inhibit neurotransmitter release. Single-dose studies resulted in a reduction in photosensitivity in all of six patients tested and there was a decrease in interictal spikes in a double-blind study with placebo and diazepam carried out in six patients. In a placebo-controlled trial of one week's duration in ten patients with refractory partial seizures, six had a greater than 50% reduction in seizures. Three double-blind studies are now in progress (Peck, 1985).

W-554

W-554 has a similar structure to the anti-anxiety agent meprobamate and exhibits a broad spectrum of anticonvulsant activity in animal models. In an open study, eight patients received W-554 as add-on therapy for 36 days. Four of these patients had a greater than 50% reduction in seizures. However, three of them had a significant rise in background anticonvulsant concentrations (Wilensky *et al.*, 1986).

Other new potential anticonvulsants include denzimol, nafimidone, saiko-keishi-to (a Chinese herbal drug) and SL 78424–00. These compounds are all effective in animal models of epilepsy and have been used in small open trials in patients with refractory epilepsy.

DERIVATIVES OF PRE-EXISTING DRUGS

Oxcarbazepine

Oxcarbazepine is the 10-keto derivative of carbamazepine. Clinical studies suggest that it might be slightly more effective and have fewer side-effects compared with carbamazepine (Houtkooper *et al.*, 1984).

CONVENTIONAL DRUGS WITH POSSIBLE ANTICONVULSANT ACTIONS

Allopurinol

Anecdotal case reports suggested that allopurinol might have anticonvulsant actions. In order to test this theory, an open study using allopurinol (250–300 mg/day) was undertaken in 40 patients, both adults and children, with refractory epilepsy. After 20 to 35 days a reduction in seizure frequency was observed, and by three to nine months 47% had a greater than 50% reduction in seizures. A multicentre double-blind study is at present in progress (De Marco and Zagnoni, 1985).

CONCLUSIONS

Since the introduction of sodium valproate more than a decade ago, no new major anticonvulsant drug has been studied clinically until recently. The availability of effective marketed antiepileptic agents made it questionable whether a new drug could capture a large enough market to justify the cost of its development, especially as many clinicians believed that improvement in seizure control depended predominantly on better utilization of existing drugs. However, the realization that a proportion of patients continue to have seizures, despite optimal use of available anticonvulsants, and that there is a need for less toxic drugs has led to renewed interest in the development of an anticonvulsant screening and drug development programme in the USA. This, coupled with recent advances in our understanding of the neurochemical basis of epilepsy and the actions of anticonvulsant drugs now in use, has led to the development of more than ten new putative anticonvulsant agents which are undergoing clinical trials at present.

Two major avenues in the future development of new anticonvulsants are possible; the first is to continue with the screening of all newly synthesized compounds; the second, which is more promising, is to develop drugs derived from a greater understanding of the pathophysiological events underlying seizure activity. Impaired inhibitory action, excessive excitatory input and abnormalities of one or more membrane ionic mechanisms may all contribute to the paroxysmal depolarizing shift of neuronal membrane potential and associated burst discharge underlying seizure activity; pharmacological manipulation is possible in all three areas. Enhancement of inhibitory actions via the GABAergic system has already led to the development of new drugs such as progabide and vigabatrin. Studies on mechanisms for decreasing excitatory neurotransmission have begun and selective antagonists of N-methyl-D-aspartate look promising in animal models of epilepsy (Meldrum, 1983). Therefore we can look forward to the availability of many new types of anticonvulsant drugs during the next decade.

REFERENCES

BINNIE, C. D., DE BEUKELAAR, F., MEIJER, J. W., MEINARDI, H., OVERWEG, J., WAUQUIER, A. and VAN WIERINGEN, A. (1985) Open dose ranging trial of flunarizine as add-on therapy in epilepsy. *Epilepsia*, **26**, 424–428.

CHADWICK, D. W. and CRAWFORD, P. M. (1986) What is epilepsy? Clinical, biochemical and pharmacological factors in seizures. In: *What is Epilepsy?*, M. Trimble and E. H. Reynolds (Eds), Churchill Livingstone, Edinburgh, pp. 53–66.

CHAPMAN, A. G. RILEY, K., EVANS, M. C. and MELDRUM, B. S. (1982) Acute effects of sodium valproate and γ-vinyl GABA on regional amino acid metabolism in the rat brain. Incorporation of (^{14}C)-glucose into amino acids. *Neurochem. Res*, **7**, 1089–1105.

CHOUSA, C., CAOMANO, J. L., ALIJANATI, R., SCARAMELLI, A., DE MEDINA, O. and ROMERO, S. (1986) Parkinsonism, tardive dyskinesia, akathisia and depression induced by flunarizine. *Lancet*, **i**, 1303–1304.

CRAWFORD, P. M. and CHADWICK, D. W. (1986) A single blind crossover comparison of progabide, valproate and placebo as add-on therapy in patients with refractory epilepsy. *J. Neurol. Neurosurg. Psychiatry*, **49**, 1251–1257.

CRAWFORD, P., GHADIALI, E., LANE, R., BLUMHARDT, L. and CHADWICK, D. (1987) Gabapentin as an epileptic drug in man. *J. Neurol. Neurosurg. Psychiatry* (in press).

DAM, M., GRAM, L., PHILBERT, A., HANSEN, B. S., BLATT LYON, B., CHRISTENSEN, J. M. and ANGELO, H. R. (1983) Progabide: a controlled trial in partial epilepsy. *Epilepsia*, **24**, 127–134.

DE MARCO, P. and ZAGNONI, P. (1985) Allopurinol and severe epilepsy. Abstract, 16th Epilepsy International Congress, Hamburg, 1985.

GIBSON, J. P. (1985) Animal safety studies with vigabatrin. Abstract, Vigabatrin in Epilepsy Symposium. Merrell Dow Research Institute.

GRAM, L., KLOSTERKOV, P. and DAM, M. (1985) Gamma-vinyl GABA: a double-blind placebo-controlled trial in partial epilepsy. *Ann. Neurol.*, **17**, 262–266.

HOUTKOOPER, M., VAN OORSCHOT, A. E. M. and HOPPENER, R. J. E. A. (1984) Oxcarbazepine (GP47.680) versus carbamazepine: A double-blind crossover study in patients with epilepsy. *Acta Neurol. Scand.*, **70**, 221.

JUNG, M. J., LIPPERT, B., METCALF, B. W., BOHLEN, B. and SCHECTER, P. J. (1977) γ-vinyl GABA (4-amino-hex-5-enoic acid), a new selective irreversible inhibitor of GABA-T: effects on brain GABA metabolism in mice. *J. Neurochem.*, **29**, 797–802.

KOIVISTO, K., SIVENIUS, J., KERNANEN, T., PARLANEN, J., RIEKKINEN, P., GOTHIONI, G., TOKOLO, O. and NEUVONEN, P. Y. (1986) Clinical trial with an experimental taurine derivative taltrimide in epileptic patients. *Epilepsia*, **27**, 87–90.

KULAKOWSKI, S., MEYNCHENS, M. and COUPEZ-LOPINOT, R. (1985) Double-blind study of a new antiepileptic drug, progabide, in severe childhood epilepsy. In: *Epilepsy and GABA Receptor Agonists*, vol. 3, G. Barthiolini *et al.* (Eds), Raven Press, New York, pp. 377–387.

LOISEAU, P., BOSSI, L., GUYOT, M., OROFIAMVNA, B. and MORSELLI, P. L. (1983) Double-blind crossover trial of progabide versus placebo in severe epilepsies. *Epilepsia*, **24**, 703–715.

MARTINEZ-LAGE, M., MORALES, G., MARTINEZ VILA, E. and POLANOS, H. (1984) Progabide treatment in severe epilepsy: a double-blind crossover trial versus placebo. *Epilepsia*, **25**, 586–593.

MELDRUM, B. (1983) Pharmacological considerations in the search for new anticonvulsant drugs. In: *Recent Advances in Epilepsy*, T. A. Pedley and B. W. Meldrum (Eds), Churchill Livingstone, Edinburgh, pp. 75–92.

OVERWEG, J., BINNIE, C. D., MEIJER, J. W., MEINARDI, H., NUIJTEN, S. T., SCHMALZ, S. and WAUQUIER, A. (1984) Double-blind placebo-controlled trial of flunarizine as add-on therapy in epilepsy. *Epilepsia*, **25**, 217–222.

PALMINTERI, R., HERITIER, C. L. and BOSSI, L. (1985) Progabide and liver function tests. Abstract, 16th Epilepsy International Congress, Hamburg, 1985.

PECK, A. W. (1985) Lamotrigine (BW430C): a new potential anticonvulsant. Abstract, 16th Epilepsy International Congress, Hamburg, 1985.

RIMMER, E. M. and RICHENS, A. (1984) Double-blind study of γ-vinyl GABA in patients with refractory epilepsy. *Lancet*, **i**, 189–190.

SACHELLARES, J. C., DONOFRIO, P. D., WAGNER, J. G., ABOU-KHALIL, B., BERENT, S. and AASVED-HOYT, K. (1985) Pilot study of zonisamide (1,2-benzisoxazole-3-methanesulfonamide) in patients with refractory partial seizures. *Epilepsia*, **26**, 206–211.

SCHMIDT, D. and UTECH, K. (1985) Progabide as adjunctive therapy in patients with complex partial seizures refractory to high-dose antiepileptic drugs. In: *Epilepsy and GABA Receptor Agonists*, vol. 3, G. Barthiolini *et al.* (Eds), Raven Press, New York, pp. 363–367.

SEINO, M. A. (1985) A collaborative clinical trial of zonisamide patients with refractory seizures. Abstract, 16th Epilepsy International Congress, Hamburg, 1985.

SPERO, L. (1982) Neurotransmitters and CNS disease: epilepsy. *Lancet*, **ii**, 1319–1322.

VAN PARYS, J. A. P., VAN DER LINEN, G. J., GOEDHART, D. M., MEIJER, J. W. A. and MEINARDI, G. J. (1985) Clinical experience with progabide in severe in- and outpatients. In: *Epilepsy and GABA Receptor Agonists*, vol. 3, G. Barthiolini *et al.* (Eds), Raven Press, New York, pp. 343–352.

WEBER, M., VERSPIGNANI, H., REMY, M. C., REGNIER, F. and BOSSI, L. (1985) Controlled trial of progabide versus placebo in severe therapy-resistant epilepsies. In: *Epilepsy and GABA Receptor Agonists*, vol. 3, G. Barthiolini *et al.* (Eds), Raven Press, New York, pp. 353–365.

WILENSKY, A. J., FRIEL, P. N., OJEMANN, L. M., DODRILL, C. B., MCCORMICK, K. B. and LEVY, R. H. (1985) Zonisamide in epilepsy; a pilot study. *Epilepsia*, **26**, 212–220.

WILENSKY, A. J., FRIEL, P. N., OJEMANN, L. H. KUPFERBERG, H. J. and LEVY, R. H. (1986) Pharmacokinetics of W-554 (ADD03055) in epileptic patients. *Epilepsia*, **26**, 602–606.

YAGI, K., NUMATA, Y., SEINO, M. and WADA, T. (1985) Pharmacokinetic parameters of zonisamide (AD810) in healthy volunteers and an open clinical trial on 30 patients with refractory seizures. Abstract, 16th Epilepsy International Congress, Hamburg, 1985.

DISCUSSION

Dr M. J. Brodie (Glasgow): It's interesting that the same things crop up repeatedly in discussion of drug action. Flunarizine, for example, though not a classical calcium antagonist, does have calcium-channel-blocking properties, as does phenytoin at high dosage. Enzyme inhibition is another recurring theme. Allopurinol reduces the metabolism of several other drugs. Verapamil and diltiazem which both control 'cardiac epilepsy' (dysrhythmias) also inhibit carbamazepine metabolism substantially. Yet they were not previously recognized as being enzyme inhibitors, although verapamil has been on the market for about 20 years. There is growing evidence that other drugs, such as cyclosporin, inhibit the activity of certain enzymes. It is important, in view of these findings, to consider the possible interactions before starting 'add-on' studies. We are now investigating the effect of nifedipine, which does not inhibit carbamazepine metabolism, in patients with intractable epilepsy. A number of them have stopped fitting but the study is not controlled. Certainly the theoretical advantages of such drugs lie in the fact that they are not psychoactive.

Crawford: In the studies with flunarizine there were no changes in background anticonvulsant therapy.

Epilepsy in Young People
Edited by E. Ross, D. Chadwick and R. Crawford

11

Temporal lobectomy in young people*

C. B. T. ADAMS
Department of Neurosurgery, Radcliffe Infirmary, Oxford

SUMMARY

Temporal lobectomy is rarely performed at present, although it is applicable to many children who could thereby be cured of their fits. Focal lesions in the brain can be located and removed by modern surgical techniques irrespective of the presence of bitemporal independent spikes. A patient is reported who had a small oligodendroglioma resected with the temporal lobe, which restored complete normality. It should be borne in mind that any surgical procedure may stop the fits for several months, but adequate follow-up for at least a year is necessary to check the results. In our series of 81 temporal lobectomy patients, more than half have obtained complete relief from their seizures. The four grades of classification were: I. complete freedom from seizures; II. up to three awake seizures per year; III. more than three overt seizures per year; IV. seizure activity greater than 10% of the pre-operative state. The overall results one year after operation were 58% of patients grade I, 11.5% grade II, 11.5% grade III and 19% grade IV. The proportion of patients who were without convulsions at one year, 58%, fell to 50% at years 3–5.

INTRODUCTION

Only a small number of children with epilepsy are suitable for surgical treatment, but there are many who could be cured of their fits who have not even been considered for surgery. Why is this? There are two main reasons. First, the view that surgery is complex, dangerous, difficult, lengthy and uncertain in its results;

*Prepared for Portsmouth symposium but not presented due to last-minute emergency.

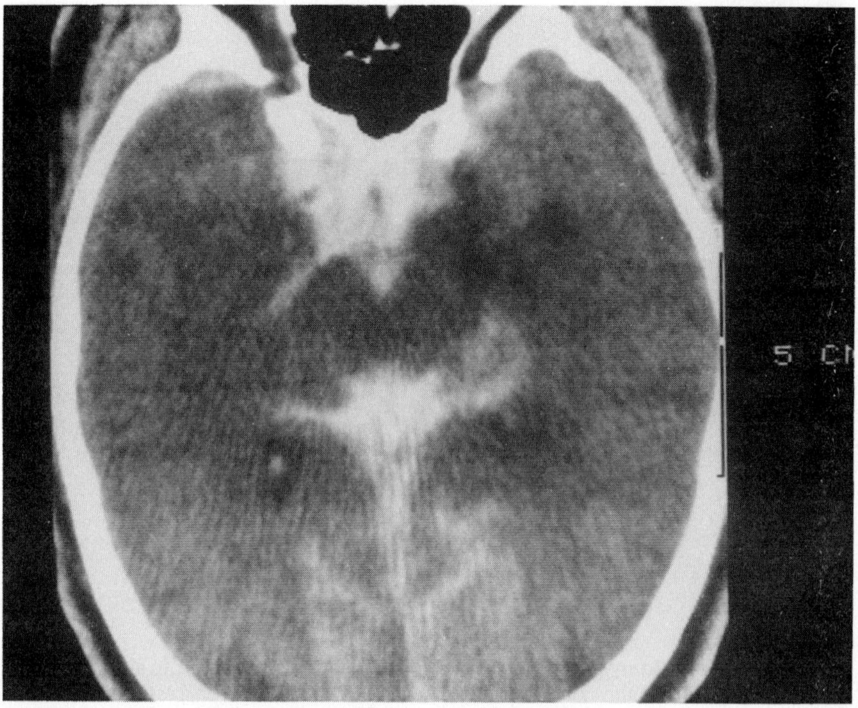

Fig. 1 Focal pathology: CT scan with intrathecal contrast medium, showing right temporal lobe tumour

people are unhappy about the many types of surgical procedures recommended in the past, and few neurosurgeons now undertake or understand surgical treatment of epilepsy. Second, the nebulous concept of excising epileptogenic cortex; there is a commonly held view that surgery merely substitutes one lesion for another.

Surgical treatment of epilepsy has, however, come of age. Nowadays, it aims to find and remove focal pathology (Fig. 1). Of course, a surgical scar is left behind, but a clean surgical scar is not in itself epileptogenic in most people. The concept of finding 'epileptogenic cortex' with a view to removing it, 'spike chasing' as it has been called, is misguided. The results are not satisfactory, and this dated approach engenders suspicion among paediatricians and neurologists, which prevents children who could be cured of their epilepsy from being referred for surgery.

That the correct aim is to remove pathology, rather than 'spikes', is illustrated by the case of a young man who had been turned down for epilepsy surgery because of bitemporal independent spiking activity. He was 16 at the time and his epilepsy had started at the age of 11. His behaviour was causing severe difficulties at home and both his social and academic prospects appeared bleak. The skull X-ray revealed a tiny speck of calcification in the right temporal lobe and I took the view that this represented a focal lesion which should be removed, irrespective of the presence of bitemporal independent spikes. A small oligodendroglioma was resected with the temporal lobe. Since the operation he has had no seizures. He is off all medication and has gone to university, obtained a degree and married. The first postoperative EEG, some three weeks after the operation, showed that the so-called 'independent spiking' in the opposite temporal lobe had completely disappeared.

One problem in assessing the results of surgery for epilepsy is that any surgical procedure may stop the fits for some months. Adequate follow-up for at least one year is therefore necessary to evaluate the results (Fig. 2). In this respect and others, finding and removing focal pathology has stood the test of time, in contrast to all other neurosurgical procedures.

RESULTS OF TEMPORAL LOBECTOMY

Among 81 temporal lobectomy patients, there has been no mortality, and more than half the patients have obtained complete freedom from their seizures. The results are classed in four grades:

I. Complete freedom from seizures.
II. Up to three awake seizures per year and/or occasional 'feelings' and/or sleep convulsions.
III. More than three overt seizures per year, but not more than 10% of pre-operative seizure activity.
IV. More than 10% of pre-operative seizure activity.

The overall results one year after operation show that 58% of patients are in grade I, 11.5% in grade II, 11.5% in grade III and 19% in grade IV. Analysis according to pathology is more informative, 68% of patients with Ammon's horn sclerosis and 76% of those with small indolent gliomas being classed as grade I. Where no focal lesion was found (in six out of 69 patients) 33% were classed as grade III, and 67% as grade IV; there were no grade I or II results. The proportion of patients without convulsions at one year, 58%, fell to 50% at years 3–5. However, 70% were in grades I and II combined at one year and this rose to 80% at years 3–5.

These bare statistics fail to convey the real effect of terminating a child's fits because disruptive behaviour always improves too, in my experience. For the first time, the brothers and sisters can bring their friends home, and parents can lead a normal life together for the first time for many years. The whole family benefits and it is little wonder that these are some of my most grateful patients.

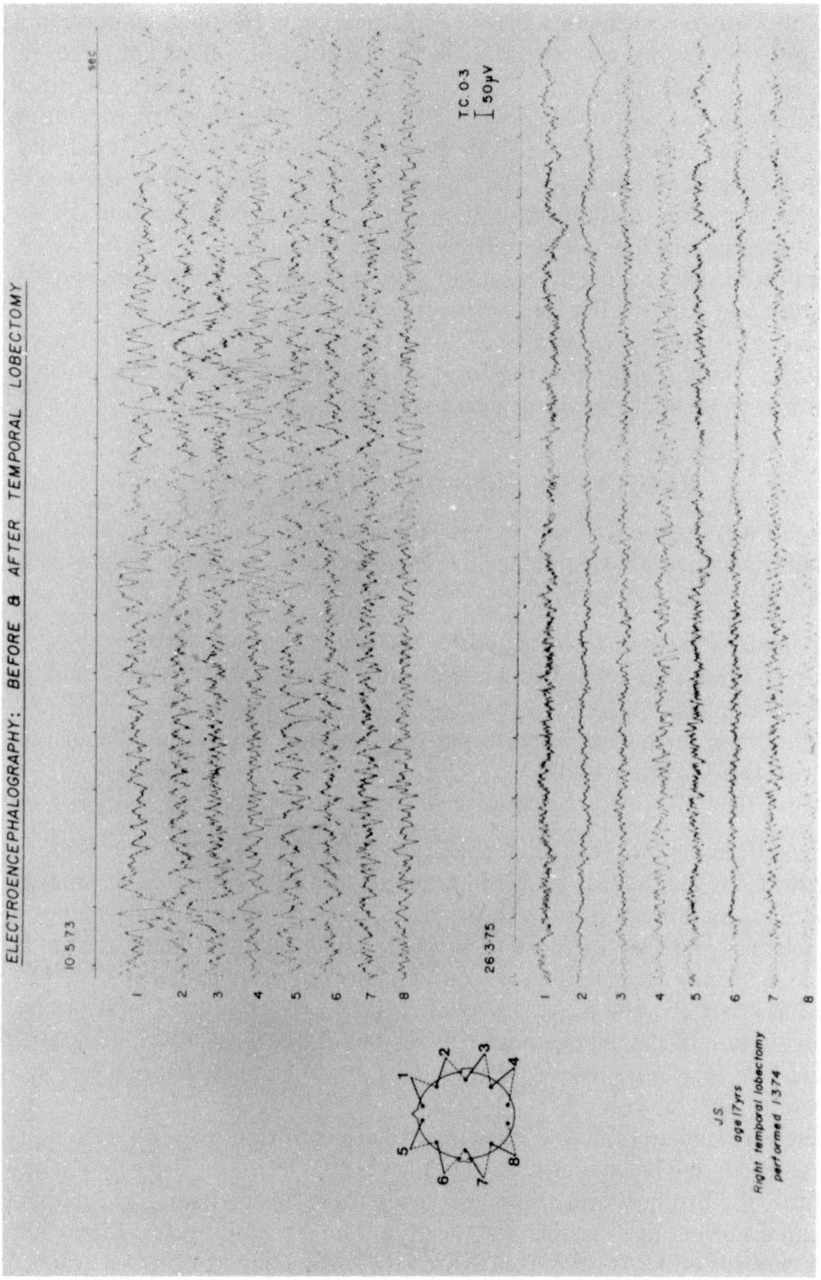

Fig. 2 EEG tracings before and one year after unilateral temporal lobectomy, showing the disappearance of temporal spikes.

SELECTION OF PATIENTS

There are four ways of looking for focal pathology in any type of epilepsy:

1. The history of the initial epileptic attack.
2. The nature of the present epileptic attacks.
3. The EEG.
4. Radiology.

History

We have learned the importance of taking a careful history of the first attack and obtaining the hospital notes where they exist. The onset of Ammon's horn sclerosis seems to be associated with a prolonged febrile convulsion between the ages of two and four years. Careful questioning often reveals that there was a temporary hemiparesis following the first convulsion, which provides useful evidence of lateralization. Ammon's horn sclerosis, curiously unilateral, often comes out of the blue with a febrile convulsion, and appears to be a minor form of infantile hemiplegia, again a condition that is curiously unilateral and sometimes amenable to hemispherectomy. The age of onset is also of importance. While Ammon's horn sclerosis starts with a prolonged febrile convulsion between two and four years of age, indolent gliomas commonly begin to cause epilepsy around eight or nine years of age, although it is likely that these tumours have been present since birth.

Nature of the attacks

The types of epileptic attack are important to analyse. We place great importance on their constancy, it being particularly helpful if the attacks always start in the same way. It does not seem to matter if the attacks then proceed differently, in form or severity. A consistent initial phase suggests that there may be a single focal origin for the epilepsy, whereas multiple fits each starting and continuing in different ways make a focal origin less probable.

EEG

The EEG is a most important tool for demonstrating the presence of a focal lesion, and is particularly helpful in the temporal and frontal lobes. The recording needs to be done carefully, and sphenoidal leads are essential. It is also extremely important to do sleep or barbiturate recordings.

Radiology

The CT scan has become the method of choice, but it too has to be done properly. Most scans are not done parallel to the temporal horn, as they should be, with the result that any lesion is obscured by the surrounding bones and the temporal horns cannot be clearly delineated. We take particular care to angle the gantry of the scanner so that the plane of the scan is parallel to the temporal horn. Various abnormalities should be sought, notably compression, distortion or dilatation of the temporal horn. Changes of density in the temporal lobe and distortion of the suprasellar cistern and Sylvian fissure are also important. In addition to specially-oriented CT scans, it may be necessary to perform scans with intravenous contrast and occasionally with intrathecal contrast media (to show up the suprasellar cistern).

TIMING OF SURGERY

Assuming the clinical features and investigations show evidence of focal pathology, often revealed as Ammon's horn sclerosis or a glioma, the next question is when to operate. In general, the answer is as soon as one is sure of the localization, for it is important to stop a child's epilepsy as soon as possible to promote full rehabilitation into society. Too many children with epilepsy still become social recluses as well as failing to achieve their potential in school due to the frequency of their subclinical and clinical fits. But how severe should the epilepsy be before surgery is considered? Standard articles almost always begin with the statement that surgery should be considered for severe frequent fits, refractory to prolonged medical treatment. But if a patient has focal pathology the epilepsy is unlikely to stop spontaneously or with medical treatment. One fit a month or one every six months will stop an adolescent driving legally and limit his education both academically and socially. Moreover, the indolence of a small so-called 'indolent' glioma cannot be guaranteed.

Surgery stops convulsions in 50–60% of patients in whom a focal lesion is found and removed. It markedly reduces the frequency in another 20%, often to just nocturnal epilepsy. Very compelling reasons are needed for not advising temporal lobectomy when a focal lesion has been found. One such consideration is whether the lesion affects the dominant temporal lobe. We know that temporal lobectomy for an indolent glioma gives rise to a verbal learning difficulty if the dominant lobe is removed, though it does not follow temporal lobectomy for Ammon's horn sclerosis. We carry out careful psychological testing in these patients, and if there is doubt about the dominant side we carry out carotid amytal testing. If a child is found to have an indolent glioma in the dominant temporal lobe, causing infrequent epilepsy, one might argue for delaying surgery until after any crucial events in the school calendar, such as important examinations.

TEMPORAL LOBECTOMY

The operation requires broad exposure, which can be obtained by a curving incision almost entirely within the hairline (Fig. 3). It entails a 6 cm en bloc

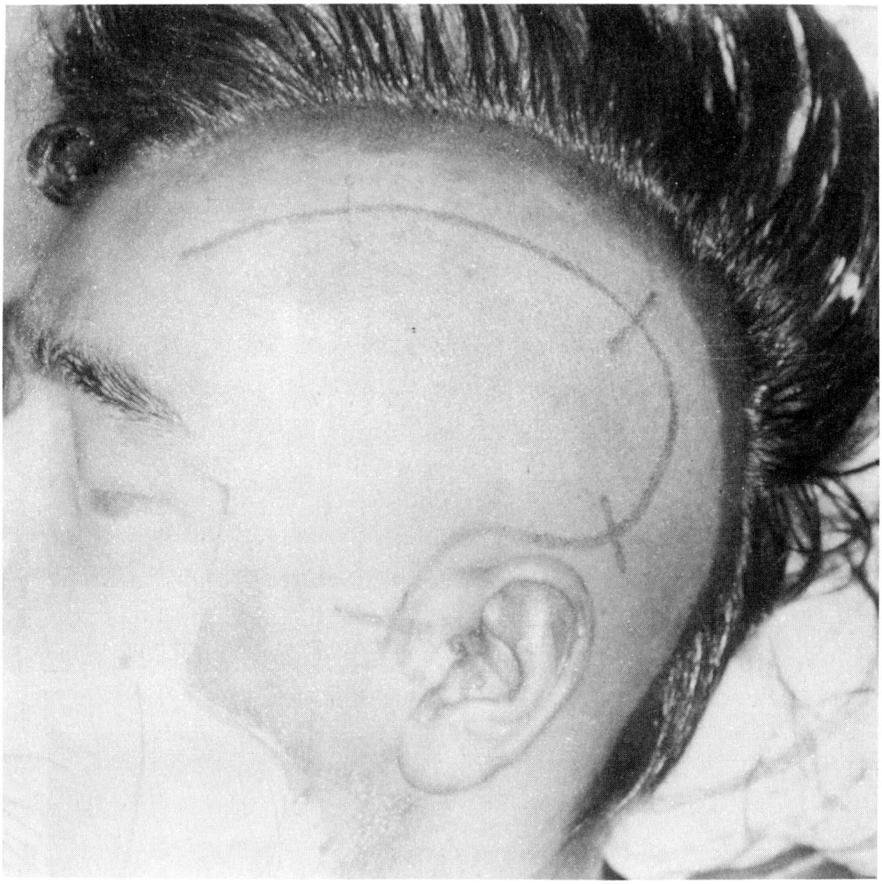

Fig. 3 Incision for temporal lobectomy

removal of the temporal lobe, which inevitably causes an upper quadrant field defect, but this is usually not apparent to the patient. (A larger resection than 6 cm causes hemianopia and, on the dominant side, dysphasia.) The operation is done under general anaesthesia, and electrocorticography is not used as all the necessary decisions have been made pre-operatively. There is one curious feature about the temporal lobe, as opposed to other parts of the cerebral hemispheres: it is important to remove the amygdala and hippocampus (Fig. 4) in addition to the local pathology (Fig. 5). This may be explained in part by the occasional finding of two lesions, one in the temporal cortex and the other, Ammon's horn sclerosis, in the hippocampus (possibly secondary to the fits induced by the first lesion when young). It does appear that the amygdala and hippocampus are structures necessary for the generation of temporal lobe

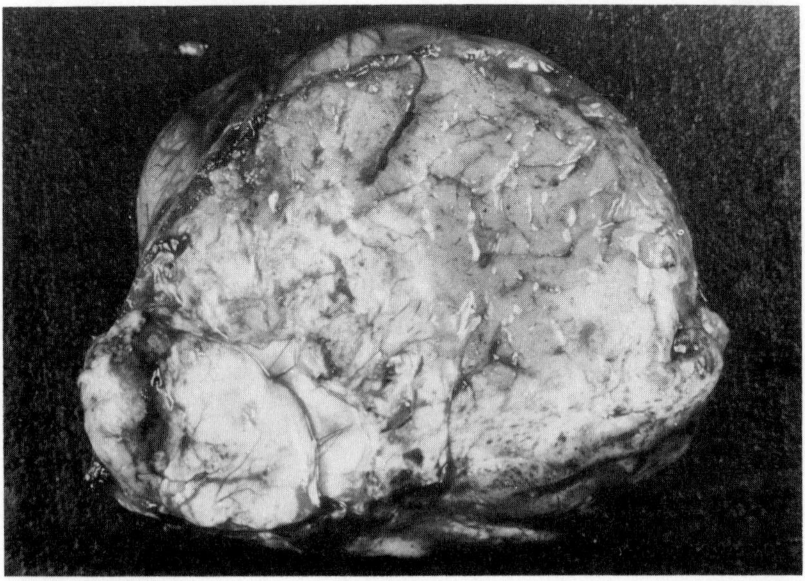

Fig. 4 Temporal lobectomy specimen showing temporal horn and hippocampus

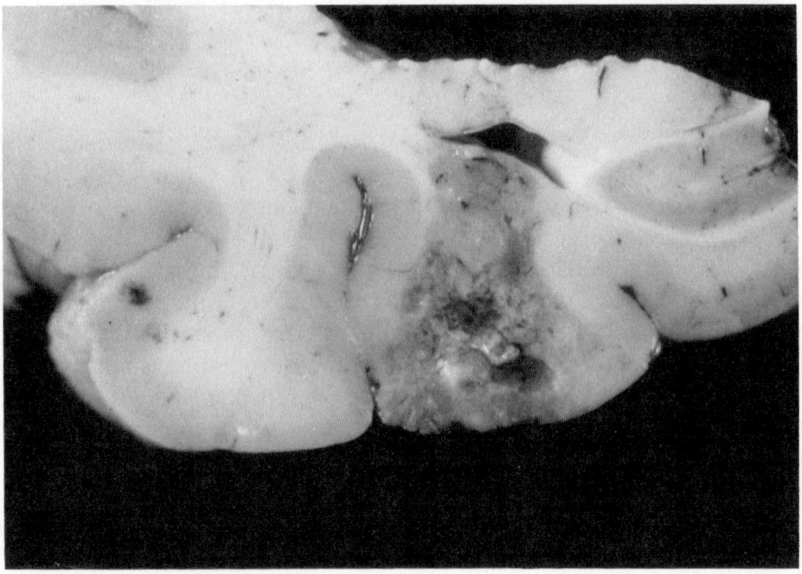

Fig. 5 Section through operation specimen showing temporal lobe tumour

epilepsy, for even if the standard temporal lobectomy fails to remove all the lesion the epilepsy may well cease post-operatively.

ACKNOWLEDGEMENT

The epilepsy surgery programme at Oxford is a team effort but I wish particularly to acknowledge the help of my neurological colleage Dr John Oxbury.

Epilepsy in Young People
Edited by E. Ross, D. Chadwick and R. Crawford

12

Selecting the appropriate therapy

SHEILA J. WALLACE
University Hospital of Wales, Cardiff

SUMMARY

The diagnosis of epilepsy in children and adolescents is usually made when the patient has had at least two seizures and probably three or more. The selection of appropriate therapy therefore is based on a confirmed diagnosis, plus an accurate identification of the type of seizure disorder. Initial medication should consist of monotherapy, weighing possible side-effects of anticonvulsant therapy against the expected benefits to the patient.

Girls with epilepsy should be made aware that their therapy may have to be continued into the reproductive period, and due consideration should be given to the possible teratogenic effects of antiepileptic drugs.

INTRODUCTION

The type of seizure disorder present is the single most important deciding factor in the selection of appropriate therapy for epilepsy in young people. For some types of epilepsy, drug therapy is not indicated. For others it may be justifiable to try all available antiepileptic medications, singly or in combination, in an attempt to obtain seizure control. In this review, the epileptic syndromes of older children and adolescents are classified as suggested by Roger *et al.* (1985). Following a brief note on the characteristics of each syndrome, the appropriate management is considered.

Unless the circumstances surrounding a first seizure are particularly compelling, it is usual to allow the patient to have two or three seizures before commencing medication. If possible monotherapy should be used. Possible side-effects from therapy must be weighed against the expected benefit to the patient. For example, it is unkind to place an adolescent girl on phenytoin, and thus risk unsightly gum hyperplasia, unless phenytoin is the only effective anticonvulsant. Therapy started in late childhood or adolescence may still be needed in early adulthood and due consideration should be given to possible teratogenic effects.

GENERALIZED EPILEPSIES

Childhood absence epilepsy (petit mal)

Childhood absence epilepsy is a form of primary generalized epilepsy which occurs predominantly in girls, with a peak age of onset between six and seven years (Loiseau, 1985a). There is a strong genetic predisposition. This syndrome begins with absence seizures, but 40% of affected children later develop generalized tonic-clonic seizures (Loiseau, 1985b). The absences occur very frequently throughout the day and may take a number of different forms (Penry *et al.*, 1975). Mild clonic components, increase or decrease in postural tone and automatisms have been observed. On the EEG absences are always associated with bilateral synchronous, symmetrical 3 Hz spike-wave discharges occurring against normal background activity. In most children absences remit about the time of puberty.

In 80% of cases absences are responsive to either ethosuximide or valproate. These two drugs are equally efficacious when used as monotherapy (Callaghan *et al.*, 1982; Sato *et al.*, 1982). In children whose absences are not complicated by generalized tonic-clonic seizures, ethosuximide is preferred. When generalized tonic-clonic seizures are also present, valproate is the drug of choice. Where neither ethosuximide nor valproate controls the absences when used alone, both together will sometimes be effective. In the small minority of patients who fail to respond to ethosuximide, valproate, or both, clonazepam is usually helpful, but tolerance is often a problem (Sato *et al.*, 1977).

Epilepsy with myoclonic absences

In epilepsy with myoclonic absences the seizures occur daily. They commence at about seven years and are more common in boys. The child is usually neurologically normal prior to the onset of myoclonic absences which are characterized by clonic jerks, which are diffuse and repeated rhythmically in relation to the 3 Hz spike-waves seen concurrently on the EEG. Tonic contractions are frequently associated with these seizures. Isolated generalized spike-waves may be noted in addition to those occurring in 3Hz runs, but the EEG background is usually normal (Tassinari, 1985). Tonic-clonic seizures present in 20% of cases and there is a tendency to evolution to other epilepsies with poor prognoses. Mental deterioration is common.

Myoclonic absences are much less responsive to therapy than other absences. Treatment with both ethosuximide and valproate controls the attacks in about half the patients, and in others diones and benzodiazepines combined with valproate may be effective.

Juvenile absence epilepsy

Absences which are clinically similar to those in childhood may commence about puberty (Wolf, 1985a). They occur infrequently, less than daily, and sporadically. Generalized tonic-clonic seizures are also present in over 80% of patients and usually occur on awakening. On the EEG, the background activity is usually normal, with the ictal discharge consisting of generalized symmetrical spike-waves with frontal accentuation. The frequency of the repetitive spike-waves is usually 3.5 to 4 Hz, i.e. rather more rapid than in other absence epilepsies. The treatment of choice in juvenile absence epilepsy is sodium valproate.

Juvenile myoclonic epilepsy

Juvenile myoclonic epilepsy commences in time-relation to puberty and is characterized by attacks in which bilateral, single or repetitive, arrhythmic, irregular myoclonic jerks involve mainly the arms (Wolf, 1985b). The seizures are virtually restricted to times of wakening from sleep, but may be precipitated by sleep deprivation. Consciousness is retained. Additional generalized tonic-clonic seizures are common. During the attacks the EEG shows rapid, generalized, repetitive spike-waves which may be irregular or take the form of polyspike-waves. Clinical accompaniments to the EEG changes are not always evident and the myoclonic jerks may not be synchronous with the EEG abnormalities. Photosensitivity is commonly present.

Valproate is the treatment of choice for juvenile myoclonic epilepsy (Asconapé and Penry, 1984; Wolf, 1985b). Primidone and phenobarbitone have also been used successfully. Even after several years of freedom from seizures while on medication, there is a high risk of relapse if therapy is discontinued (Asconapé and Penry, 1984; Wolf, 1985b).

Progressive myoclonic epilepsy in childhood and adolescence

Progressive myoclonic epilepsy (PME) presents clinically in one of the following ways: a myoclonic syndrome associating generalized myoclonus with arrhythmic, asynchronous and asymmetrical, partial or segmental, myoclonus; an epileptic syndrome in which the seizures are of various types, the most frequent being generalized tonic-clonic, myoclonic and tonic; a progressive mental deterioration leading to dementia; and abnormal cerebellar, pyramidal, and later, extrapyramidal signs on neurological examination (Roger, 1985). The EEG shows progressive deterioration of background rhythms; spikes, spike-wave or generalized spike-wave activity; and progressive disorganization of sleep-patterns. Identifiable causes of PME are juvenile Gaucher's disease, Spielmeyer–Vogt–Sjögren disease, and Lafora's disease, but in most cases the aetiology is unknown.

Selection of the appropriate therapy for PME is clearly difficult. In some cases valproate may be helpful. If generalized tonic-clonic seizures are prominent and uncontrolled by valproate, phenytoin is worth a trial, and carbamazepine, primidone or phenobarbitone can lead to improvement in some patients. Seizure control is achieved with either clonazepam or nitrazepam, but tolerance develops rapidly and in some cases very large doses of benzodiazepines are necessary. Patients resistant to conventional antiepileptic drugs may sometimes respond to ACTH, corticosteroids or a ketogenic diet.

Epilepsy with primary generalized tonic-clonic seizures

When the epilepsy consists entirely of primary generalized tonic-clonic seizures and the EEG shows normal background activity with either no other abnormality or bilateral spike-wave, valproate, phenytoin, carbamazepine, primidone or phenobarbitone are probably equally efficacious. It is therefore important to consider the likelihood of unwanted effects. Phenytoin should be avoided in adolescents, particularly girls, since unsightly gum hyperplasia is common. Primidone and phenobarbitone are more likely than the other drugs to cause undesirable behaviour. Carbamazepine is relatively free of side-effects, but needs to be administered at least twice daily. In the case of valproate, serious side-effects are extremely rare and most likely to appear in very young, severely retarded children. On balance, valproate is the drug of first choice for primary generalized tonic-clonic seizures. Nevertheless concerns about its possible teratogenic effects remain, and for young females starting treatment in adolescence the possibility that treatment might need to be continued during pregnancy should not be ignored.

Epilepsy with generalized tonic-clonic seizures on awakening

Generalized tonic-clonic seizures occurring almost exclusively in the first two hours after awakening, but on occasions also during evening relaxation, usually have their onset during the second decade (Wolf, 1985c). If other seizures are present, they are likely to be absences or myoclonias. Increased slow waves, disorganization of background activity with steep transients and, less commonly, generalized spike-wave activity, are found on the EEG.

Sleep deficit, excessive alcohol intake and sudden external arousal predispose susceptible individuals to seizures. Avoidance of these precipitating factors is as important as drug therapy. It may be necessary for affected patients to avoid jobs entailing shift work.

About two-thirds of patients will achieve complete seizure control with attention to precipitating factors and drug therapy. Barbiturates are reported to be more effective than phenytoin or carbamazepine (Wolf, 1985c). Since valproate is particularly useful in other generalized epilepsies, it might be expected to prevent generalized tonic-clonic seizures on waking, but no trial has yet been reported.

Photosensitive epilepsies

Seizures induced by flickering lights may consist of mild clonic jerking, but are usually generalized and tonic-clonic (Jeavons and Harding, 1975). Of patients who are sensitive to intermittent photic stimuli 30% are also pattern sensitive (Wilkins and Lindsay, 1985).

Seizures induced by intermittent photic stimulation can very often be averted by physical rather than pharmaceutical methods. Television-induced seizures may be prevented by a small screen, not sitting too close, remote control for switching on and off or changing the programme; or using 'television glasses' (Wilkins and Lindsay, 1985). In other circumstances, such as light flickering on water, occlusion of the vision to one eye by using a hand, or crossed polaroid spectacles will reduce the likelihood of clinical seizure. Where physical methods do not control photosensitive epilepsy, valproate is the drug of first choice.

PARTIAL EPILEPSIES

Benign partial epilepsies of childhood

Children with benign partial epilepsies have the following clinical criteria (Dalla Bernardino, 1985). There are no intellectual or neurological deficits. A family history of benign epilepsy is common. Seizures start after the age of 18 months, are usually brief, frequent at the onset, but later rare, and respond readily to treatment. There is no prolonged deficit post-ictally and neurological and psychological development proceed normally. The EEGs are characterized by normal background activity, with focal abnormalities which, in individual patients, may consist of centro-temporal spikes, occipital paroxysms, or frontal or mid-temporal spikes. Sleep organization is normal. The EEG abnormalities are age-dependent, not associated with demonstrable anatomical changes, and recover spontaneously.

Since benign partial epilepsies of childhood are self-limiting, tending to remit at puberty, anticonvulsant therapy is not always necessary. Nevertheless, on the whole, parents prefer to have their children on medication, since this is likely to allow greater participation in unsupervised activities. Carbamazepine is the drug of first choice.

Benign partial seizures of adolescents

Benign partial seizures with onset in adolescence start at a peak of 13 to 14 years, and predominate in males of normal neurological and intellectual status with no family history of epilepsy (Loiseau and Louiset, 1985). The seizures are mainly associated with motor and/or sensory symptoms, and become secondarily generalized in about two-thirds of cases. A single seizure is the total ictal event in four-fifths of those adolescents affected; they should not be started on antiepileptic medication. For the rest, carbamazepine is the most appropriate therapy.

Partial epilepsies secondary to definable lesions

The clinical expressions of seizures secondary to anatomical abnormalities are infinitely variable, being dependent on the location of the lesion. When a definite lesion has been demonstrated medical therapy is used to the maximal levels tolerable. Phenytoin, carbamazepine, valproate and/or primidone can all be useful. If maximal dosage of one of these is unhelpful, combinations should be considered.

PARTIAL SEIZURES SECONDARILY GENERALIZED

The seizures in both benign and lesional partial epilepsies may become secondarily generalized. On the whole, therapy is better addressed to the partial onset than to the secondary generalization. Thus, carbamazepine or phenytoin would be most favoured in the first instance, with consideration given to valproate or primidone as second-line therapy.

CONCLUSIONS

Selection of the appropriate therapy for epilepsy in young people should be based on a certainty of the diagnosis, an accurate identification of the type of epilepsy, a knowledge of those classes of epilepsy which do not need drugs, an understanding of the risk-benefit balance for side-effects and anticonvulsant efficacy, and an awareness, for females, that therapy might have to continue into the reproductive period.

REFERENCES

Ascoɴapé, J. and Penry, J. K. (1984) Some clinical and EEG aspects of benign juvenile myoclonic epilepsy. *Epilepsia*, **25**, 108–114.

Callaghan, N., O'Hare, J., O'Driscoll, D., O'Neill, B. and Daly, M. (1982) Comparative study of ethosuximide and sodium valproate in the treatment of typical absence seizures (petit mal). *Dev. Med. Child Neurol.*, **24**, 830–836.

DALLA BERNARDINO, B. (1985) Benign partial epilepsies. In: *Epileptic Syndromes in Infancy, Childhood and Adolescence*, J. Roger *et al.* (Eds), John Libbey Eurotext, London, p. 322.

JEAVONS, P. M. and HARDING, G. F. A. (1975) *Photosensitive Epilepsy*, Clinics in Developmental Medicine, No. 56, Heinemann Medical, London.

LOISEAU, P. (1985a) Childhood absence epilepsy. In: *Epileptic Syndromes in Infancy, Childhood and Adolescence*, J. Roger *et al.* (Eds), John Libbey Eurotext, London, p. 312.

LOISEAU, P. (1985b) Childhood absence epilepsy. In: *Epileptic Syndromes in Infancy, Childhood and Adolescence*, J. Roger *et al.* (Eds), John Libbey Eurotext, London, pp. 106–120.

LOISEAU, P. and LOUISET, P. (1985) Benign partial seizures of adolescence. In: *Epileptic Syndromes in Infancy, Childhood and Adolescence*, J. Roger *et al.* (Eds), John Libbey Eurotext, London, pp. 274–277.

PENRY, J. K., PORTER, R. J. and DREIFUSS, F. E. (1975) Simultaneous recording of absence seizures with videotape and electroencephalography. A study of 374 seizures in 48 patients. *Brain*, **98**, 427–440.

ROGER, J. (1985) Progressive myoclonic epilepsy in childhood and adolescence. In: *Epileptic Syndromes in Infancy, Childhood and Adolescence*, J. Roger *et al.* (Eds), John Libbey Eurotext, London, pp. 302–310.

ROGER, J., DRAVET, C., BUREAU, M., DREIFUSS, F. E. and WOLF, P. (1985) *Epileptic Syndromes in Infancy, Childhood and Adolescence*, John Libbey Eurotext, London.

SATO, S., PENRY, J. K., DREIFUSS, F. E. and DYKEN, P. R. (1977) Clonazepam in the treatment of absence seizures: double-blind clinical trial. *Neurology*, **27**, 371.

SATO, S., WHITE, B. G. and PENRY, J. K. (1982) Valproic acid versus ethosuximide in the treatment of absence seizures. *Neurology*, **32**, 157–163.

TASSINARI, C. A. (1985) Epilepsy with myoclonic absences. In: *Epileptic Syndromes in Infancy, Childhood and Adolescence*, J. Roger *et al.* (Eds), John Libbey Eurotext, London, p. 321.

WILKINS, A. and LINDSAY, J. (1985) Common forms of reflex epilepsy: physiological mechanisms and techniques for treatment. In: *Recent Advances in Epilepsy*, no. 2, T. A. Pedley and B. S. Meldrum (Eds), Churchill Livingstone, London, pp. 239–271.

WOLF, P. (1985a) Juvenile absence epilepsy. In: *Epileptic Syndromes in Infancy, Childhood and Adolescence*, J. Roger *et al.* (Eds), John Libbey Eurotext, London, pp. 242–246.

WOLF, P. (1985b) Juvenile myoclonic epilepsy. In: *Epileptic Syndromes in Infancy, Childhood and Adolescence*, J. Roger *et al.* (Eds), John Libbey Eurotext, London, pp. 247–258.

WOLF, P. (1985c) Epilepsy with grand mal on awakening. In: *Epileptic Syndromes in Infancy, Childhood and Adolescence*, J. Roger *et al.* (Eds), John Libbey Eurotext, London, pp. 259–270.

PANEL DISCUSSION

Dr M. J. Brodie (Glasgow): Do you think that adult seizures can be defined as closely as childhood seizures by studying the different syndromes?

Dr S. J. Wallace (Cardiff): I can't see why not. A very large patient population would need to be divided into categories that are readily definable as epilepsy and those that are not. This may not be easy where the categories tend to overlap. For example, some of the juvenile and childhood epilepsies are not really separable: early morning myoclonic epilepsies often run together with the early morning generalized tonic-clonic attacks. The classification of childhood epilepsy is a very good attempt at defining these syndromes, but we all need to look at our own epileptic patients and see whether they fit these categories.

Dr W. H. Schutt (Bristol): Dr Brodie, you must see a great variety of women on different forms and combinations of therapy. Is your own personal preference for monotherapy and reduction in the number of drugs used?

Brodie: It really depends on what type of epilepsy the patient has, what problems they have, what drugs they are on, and what drugs they seem to have found useful. If the last drug that was added appeared to be the most helpful, it might be the one to choose. If a patient is on polypharmacy, I measure the concentrations of all the drugs, decide on one and then reduce the others by one dosage increment each month. With phenobarbitone, I sometimes continue them on a tiny dose rather than withdraw it altogether. I haven't been avoiding phenytoin specifically—or valproate—in young women if the patient appears to be benefiting substantially. Many patients on valproate have now heard of the risk of spina bifida. Nevertheless, their epilepsy may respond well to this drug which is particularly valuable for many forms of adolescent seizures. In some cases we have to live with that risk, hoping to change the treatment before pregnancy or to detect an abnormality if it occurs. The decisions have to be made very early, and perhaps we should be trying other drugs first in susceptible patients, until the position becomes clearer.

Dr D. W. Chadwick (Liverpool): For adult patients with epilepsy, there is no very good evidence of differing efficacy between the antiepileptic drugs currently available. Some patients with very benign epilepsies will do well on small doses of almost any anticonvulsant drug, whereas others will do badly no matter what drug or drugs you give them. The choice of therapy then rests largely on what is known about adverse effects, notably on cognitive functioning. For adult patients, I would usually give either valproate or carbamazepine in preference to older drugs such as phenytoin and phenobarbitone. I have very rarely used benzodiazepines in adults, yet many of the adolescent patients who come to me are taking a benzodiazepine, which is often difficult to withdraw because of the risk of withdrawal seizures. How often are benzodiazepines effective in the long-term treatment of childhood epilepsies that we adult neurologists don't see?

Dr J. Stephenson (Glasgow): This problem has not been clearly defined in relation to the epilepsies seen by paediatric neurologists and paediatricians, who are sometimes tempted to prescribe benzodiazepines in large amounts. May I pose a therapeutic problem to the panel? In what sequence and dosage should medications be prescribed for a 12-year-old with complex focal seizures every hour of the day and night, going wild and kicking and obviously requiring medication? There is no focal abnormality in the EEG, he doesn't want to spend weeks in hospital and he has come 100 miles to get treatment.

Wallace: When a child has been having many partial seizures over, say, a day or two, it is justifiable to start with carbamazepine and to put it up to a maximal dose over two to three days. The response tends to be rapid in these circumstances, usually within 24–36 hours. If there is not a good response within 48 hours, other drugs should be tried. There may be some place for short-term benzodiazepine while loading the child with say, phenytoin. With other antiepileptic drugs it is hard to know how long to wait before deciding whether it is likely to become effective, but carbamazepine has almost always solved that problem for me.

Brodie: I agree. Partly as a consequence of our autoinduction studies, I put most patients on carbamazepine for one reason or another these days; and the psychomotor side-effects also seem to favour carbamazepine. The one concern is that some patients seem to attain high concentrations quite quickly, presumably because autoinduction is less active. We therefore need to ensure that excessive blood levels do not rapidly produce psychomotor impairment, dizziness, nausea and headache. Otherwise patient confidence and cooperation may be seriously impaired. I would therefore start with a modest dose and see if there is a therapeutic effect; the patient should then be warned of possible side-effects and the dose rapidly increased. If necessary the dose can be reduced for a while, pending determination of blood levels.

Dr C. M. Verity (Cambridge): From the paediatric viewpoint, I wonder how often benzodiazepines do actually provide prolonged control of seizures? Secondly, there has been a trend towards valproate and carbamazepine as the newer and more effective, or perhaps more popular, anticonvulsants with fewer side-effects, but I wonder whether the panel feel that this trend needs re-evaluation in view of the side-effects reported during the last two or three years?

Wallace: The interesting thing about valproate is that the really serious side-effects have been mainly in children under the age of two, whose epilepsy may well be a symptom of an underlying degenerative or metabolic condition. As regards the neural tube defects that may be due to valproate, there is quite a high chance of diagnosing these early in pregnancy and taking appropriate action. Although I don't see that as being a very satisfactory way of going about things, it is a more clear-cut situation to handle than, for example, the relatively nebulous side-effects of phenytoin.

Dr M. R. Trimble (London): In drug trials we tend to ask patients how many seizures they have had, without enquiring about changes in the nature of the seizures. Yet benzodiazepines and other drugs quite often modify a patient's seizures. For example, patients who have partial seizures with complex automatisms and disturbed behaviour for ten minutes or more thereafter may have those seizures transformed into a much briefer partial seizure. This can be very important for the patient or the parents because the behaviour disturbance is minimized, but the change may not be recorded if seizures are simply counted.

Secondly, may I ask Dr Chadwick to comment on the VA study (Mattson *et al.*, 1985) of antiepileptic therapy in more than 600 patients?

Chadwick: The patients were randomized to therapy with a single drug (carbamazepine, phenytoin, phenobarbitone or primidone), and its success was measured by the percentage of patients who remained on the drug throughout the study. The findings showed that phenobarbitone and particularly primidone were less likely to be continued by patients than phenytoin and carbamazepine. The major differences between drugs were due to the adverse effects rather than differences in efficacy. Carbamazepine may also be more efficacious for complex partial seizures than phenobarbitone or primidone. However, there were some problems with the study, 200 patients being lost to follow-up within the first year without adequate explanation. As regards changes in seizure patterns, I have doubts about including this factor in drug trials. Studies of epilepsy are complicated enough as it is; we are more likely to get clear answers by asking relatively simple questions about major changes.

REFERENCE

MATTSON, R. H., CRAMER, J. A., COLLINS, J. F. *et al.* (1985) Comparison of carbamazepine, phenobarbitone, phenytoin and primidone in partial and secondarily generalized tonic-clonic seizures. *N. Engl. J. Med.*, **313**, 145–151.

Section III: New Areas of Study in Epilepsy

Epilepsy in Young People
Edited by E. Ross, D. Chadwick and R. Crawford

13

Recent developments in childhood non-convulsive status epilepticus

GREGORY STORES
National Centre for Children with Epilepsy, Park Hospital for Children, and University Department of Psychiatry, Oxford

SUMMARY

In classifying status epilepticus there is a basic distinction between convulsive and non-convulsive forms. The four non-convulsive types are: (1) secondary generalized myoclonic-astatic, (2) primary generalized myoclonic-astatic, (3) typical absence status, and (4) complex partial status. Recognition of non-convulsive status can be difficult because of the subtle ways in which the disorder may present. Clinical manifestations range from stupor, at one extreme, to minor changes such as clouding of consciousness, likely to be detected only by very careful observation or psychological testing.

Although non-convulsive status may not respond well to treatment and tends to relapse, it is clearly appropriate to try to improve the child's immediate well-being by energetic treatment in order to reduce the risk of further episodes and possible brain damage.

INTRODUCTION

For most people, 'status epilepticus' brings to mind a prolonged convulsion, carrying serious risk of brain damage, if not death, and commanding urgent attention. In fact, the term goes well beyond this dramatic situation to cover any seizure which is abnormally prolonged. In principle, there are as many types of status epilepticus as there are types of seizure (Gastaut, 1983). A basic distinction can be made between convulsive and non-convulsive forms.

Non-convulsive status has been the subject of relatively limited study. Reports have been largely sporadic, although recent reviews are beginning to provide a more comprehensive picture (Doose, 1983; Porter and Penry, 1983; Treiman and Delgado-Escueta, 1983; Stores, 1986). Various issues of considerable practical and theoretical importance have arisen from these and other reports.

Basic definitions present some difficulties, but for the present purposes status epilepticus can be defined as abnormal prolongation of a seizure, or serial repetition without full recovery between seizures. Its duration ranges from many minutes to much longer. Some patients in non-convulsive status seem to have been affected for weeks or even months.

Non-convulsive status epilepticus is essentially behavioural in manifestation without prominent or sometimes any motor manifestations. The most commonly described form of non-convulsive status is generalized or absence status of which typical and atypical varieties are distinguished. Much less commonly reported is complex partial status. Both generalized and partial non-convulsive status occur in children. It is impossible to know with what frequency, but certainly the generalized form is not the rarity once thought. Aspects of non-convulsive status in which advances are being made include: classification in children, awareness of its varied clinical presentation, and appreciation of the risk of further neurological impairment.

CLASSIFICATION OF NON-CONVULSIVE STATUS

Classification of non-convulsive status in children is probably even more difficult than classification elsewhere in the epilepsies. The aim is to make distinctions of practical value and, ideally, of neurophysiological validity. For practical purposes there is some merit in considering the following four types of childhood non-convulsive status. The first two tend to begin between the ages of one and seven years; the second two are usually described in later childhood and adolescence (Stores 1986).

Non-convulsive status in children with the Lennox–Gastaut syndrome (secondary generalized myoclonic-astatic epilepsy)

The concept of the Lennox–Gastaut syndrome is confused (Aicardi, 1973) but, in general, it is characterized by: a combination of seizure types (especially myoclonic, atonic and atypical absence seizures), diffuse slow spike-wave EEG discharges, and mental retardation. Children of this type who develop non-convulsive status are usually described as showing 'pseudodementia' and 'pseudoataxia', that is confusion, unresponsiveness, drooling of saliva and poor coordination, which is partly the result of multiple small jerks of the limbs. 'Petit mal status', 'minor motor status' and 'minor epileptic status', as well as other somewhat inappropriate terms are often used for this condition.

Non-convulsive status in a variant of the Lennox–Gastaut syndrome (primary generalized myoclonic-astatic epilepsy)

Doose (1983) has drawn attention to the apparently uncommon primary generalized myoclonic-astatic epilepsy which is like the Lennox–Gastaut syndrome in some respects but crucially different in others. In particular, it occurs mainly in non-retarded children who seem especially prone to develop non-convulsive status. The clinical picture is similar to that of typical Lennox–Gastaut patients. 'Atypical absence status' refers to this condition.

Typical absence status

This is a rare complication of absence epilepsy. Generalized, regular 3 Hz spike-wave discharge is associated with very obviously altered consciousness (Ohtahara *et al.*, 1979).

Complex partial status

This has been described mainly in adults but also occasionally in children with complex partial epilepsy. The EEG changes in this form of status can consist of localized discharges or more diffuse changes but generalized spike-wave activity is not seen. The usual clinical picture appears to be similar to that of generalized non-convulsive status, but can be much more florid.

CLINICAL PRESENTATION

Reference has already been made to the clinical changes usually reported in these various forms of non-convulsive status. Their behavioural nature often causes delay or failure to recognize non-convulsive status as an epileptic disorder because this type of epileptic manifestation is unfamiliar to many physicians. The resulting misdiagnoses include ascribing of the regressed, unresponsive or disturbed state to antiepileptic drug intoxication, prolonged postictal state, acute encephalopathy, neurodegenerative disorder or primary psychiatric cause, including depression, hysteria or psychosis. The condition may not be recognized at all in subnormal patients because of similarity with the basic handicapped state. In a recently described series (Stores, 1986) non-convulsive status had not been clinically diagnosed in ten out of twenty patients in spite of prominent clinical manifestations.

A further and serious difficulty in recognizing non-convulsive status can be attributed to the subtle ways in which it may show itself. Reports in the literature tend to have dwelt on the more dramatic manifestations described above, but it is clear that a spectrum of possible clinical change exists from stupor at one extreme to minor changes at the other, such as very mild clouding of consciousness, which require very careful observation or psychological testing for their detection. There are also striking examples of children whose prolonged seizure discharge is not apparently accompanied by any clinical change at all.

Certain general features of non-convulsive status help in its recognition. Usually (but not always) it develops in patients with a past history of epilepsy and consists of deterioration without obvious cause. The diagnosis is particularly suggested if the child equally mysteriously returns to his usual self. A standard EEG during the period of disturbance should be helpful. Long-term ambulatory cassette monitoring can be valuable for detecting repeated episodes of status, including those of very subtle manifestation (Stores, 1985).

TREATMENT

In the series of children already quoted (Stores, 1986) a further worrying finding was that in only nine of the 20 children diagnosed as having non-convulsive status had there been any vigorous attempt to treat the bout of status. Half the children seem to have continued in status for weeks and months after the diagnosis was first made.

The effects of emergency treatment are unpredictable and often disappointing. Even when a child responds to rectal diazepam or other attempts at intervention, relapse may well occur in spite of changes in continuous medication. Nevertheless, it is clearly appropriate to try to improve the child's immediate well-being by energetic treatment and to attempt to prevent further episodes of status.

RISK OF FURTHER NEUROLOGICAL IMPAIRMENT

The argument in support of such therapeutic efforts is strengthened by clinical and experimental reports which suggest that prolonged exposure to non-convulsive seizure discharge might damage the brain. This warning has been sounded particularly by Doose and his colleagues (Doose and Völzke, 1979). They report a much higher rate of later intellectual impairment in children with primary generalized myoclonic-astatic epilepsy who had suffered recurrent bouts of non-convulsive status, compared with those who have not experienced this complication.

Whether or not the brain-damaging effects of non-convulsive status as suggested by these and other reports are confirmed, this disorder is clearly to be avoided or controlled as well as possible. In general, drug treatment should follow the same lines as that for convulsive status, although much needs to be discovered about effective suppression of this intriguing and serious form of epilepsy.

REFERENCES

AICARDI, J. (1973) The problem of the Lennox syndrome. *Dev. Med. Child Neurol.*, **15**, 77–80.

DOOSE, H. (1983) Non-convulsive status epilepticus in childhood; clinical aspects and classification. In: *Advances in Neurology*, vol. 34, *Status Epilepticus*, A. V. Delgado-Escueta *et al.* (Eds), Raven Press, New York, pp. 83–92.

DOOSE, H. and VÖLZKE, E. (1979) Petit mal status in early childhood and dementia. *Neuropädiatrie*, **10**, 10–14.

GASTAUT, H. (1983) Classification of status epilepticus. In: *Advances in Neurology*, vol. 34, *Status Epilepticus*, A. V. Delgado-Escueta *et al.* (Eds), Raven Press, New York, pp. 15–35.

OHTAHARA, S., OKA, E., YAMATOGI, Y., OHTSUKA, Y., ISHIDA, T., ICHIBA, N.,it ISHIDA, S. and MIYAKE, S. (1979) Non-convulsive status epilepticus in childhood. *Folia Psychiatr. Neurol. Jpn.*, **33**, 345–351.

PORTER, R. J. and PENRY, J. K. (1983) Petit mal status. In: *Advances in Neurology*, vol. 34, *Status Epilepticus*, A. V. Delgado-Escueta (Eds), Raven Press, New York, pp. 61–67.

STORES, G. (1985) Clinical and EEG evaluation of seizures and seizure-like disorders. *J. Am. Acad. Child Psychiatry*, **24**, 10–16.

STORES, G. (1986) Non-convulsive status epilepticus in children. In: *Recent Advances in Epilepsy 3*, T. A. Pedley and B. S. Meldrum (Eds), Churchill Livingstone, Edinburgh, pp. 295–310.

TREIMAN, D. M. and DELGADO-ESCUETA, A. V. (1983) Complex partial status epilepticus. In: *Advances in Neurology*, vol. 34, *Status Epilepticus*, A. V. Delgado-Escueta *et al.* (Eds), Raven Press, New York, pp. 69–81.

DISCUSSION

Dr M. R. Trimble (London), Chairman: You didn't mention what is perhaps the most fascinating aspect of non-convulsive status, that is, the patients that show no surface electroencephalographic abnormalities.

Stores: My intention was to deal with the kind of case that might be encountered in everyday clinical practice. I presume you are referring to the rare instances in which depth-electrode recording shows changes but simultaneous scalp recordings show little, if anything.

Trimble: Exactly. This raises all sorts of issues about how you define an epileptic seizure and the associated EEG changes. Can we call something a seizure if, for example, a psychotic patient has spike-wave activity coming from the hippocampus, amygdala and septal regions of the brain? What is the relationship between such phenomena and a patient with a similar clinical presentation who has gross EEG abnormalities in the surface recording? Such cases are well documented, with marked cognitive and/or behavioural disorders (including aggressive behaviour) associated with discharges confined to the limbic system which do not show on surface EEG recordings.

Stores: Those findings raise very difficult issues, but in practice if seizures are suspected clinically then we should be prepared to make a tentative diagnosis even in the absence of EEG abnormalities on scalp recordings.

Dr E. M. Ross (London): A very interesting parallel is developing between epileptology and cardiology. Thirty years or so ago, cardiologists stopped talking in general terms about blue babies and congenital hearts and began to describe specific syndromes and make precise cardiological diagnoses. New technologies make this possible, not only by providing novel means of investigation, but also be revealing characteristic signs, some of which could then be detected clinically. In epilepsy too, it is now becoming possible to make clinical diagnoses because more is known as a result of more sophisticated investigations. The tragedy is that so many children are still not diagnosed earlier. A meeting like this could demonstrate that more sophisticated epilepsy diagnoses *can* now be made. It is time to stop talking about a child having 'epilepsy' and make a precise diagnosis in each case. How can we get this educational point across to the profession? Is it worth printing a checklist for the sort of epilepsies that ought to be considered whenever a child is suspected of having seizures?

Stores: The essential requirement is to encourage all concerned to describe *exactly* what happens in attacks. This may seem very obvious, but often it isn't done; people too readily opt for ambiguous terms like grand mal and petit mal. A precise description is needed of what happens, subjectively and objectively, together with the circumstances in which attacks occur. Given that sort of detailed clinical information, the vital distinctions to which you are referring start to come to light.

Dr J. Stephenson (Glasgow): Why don't you advise steroids for serious status?

Stores: The list of treatments I gave was meant to indicate first-line approaches, but there are quite a few of these children, perhaps especially the retarded ones, who may need a whole range of treatments including steroids but with variable response.

Dr R. McWilliam (Stirling): Do you think infantile spasms can be seen as a form of non-convulsive status?

Stores: Yes, in some cases at least. You would need to demonstrate that an infant's responsiveness was diminished during the hypsarrhythmic period, which might be very difficult to establish especially in retarded infants.

Epilepsy in Young People
Edited by E. Ross, D. Chadwick and R. Crawford

14

Ambulatory EEG monitoring: a preliminary follow-up study

T. E. POWELL (Speaker), G. F. A. HARDING and P. M. JEAVONS
Clinical Neurophysiology Unit, Department of Vision Sciences, Aston University, Birmingham

SUMMARY

Ambulatory monitoring in children is particularly useful for recording the frequency and pattern of occurrence of absence seizures and the response to medication. It is also used to help differentiate attacks of an uncertain nature and to clarify the type of seizure. An analysis of our first 215 recordings showed that just over half the patients referred for ambulatory monitoring were under the age of 21 years. Of patients who experienced attacks, a positive diagnosis of epilepsy was more often made in children (50%) than in adults (22%). Just under half the children whose attacks showed no EEG abnormality were being treated with anticonvulsants. A follow-up study of these children showed that half were no longer receiving anticonvulsant therapy and that their attacks had ceased. Half were still being treated and in four of these the final diagnosis was epilepsy.

INTRODUCTION

Ambulatory EEG monitoring has been employed increasingly in the diagnosis of epilepsy over the last ten years. The small portable four- and eight-channel cassette recorders enable patients to be monitored for several days in their normal environment, so that EEG sampling time is increased and attacks are more likely to be recorded. The technique has been used to aid in differentiation of epileptic and non-epileptic attacks, to quantify seizure discharges in patients with absences, to assess the effect of the environment on attacks and to record sleep in patients outside the laboratory.

To obtain the greatest advantage from the technique it should be used on patients whose attacks are sufficiently frequent to occur at least once during the period of recording. Although sometimes the sleep EEG may provide useful information the basal waking EEG is often unrevealing, and the interpretation of interictal abnormalities can be difficult particularly in children. We record mainly from patients who experience at least one attack a week and we ensure that there is the possibility of prolonging recordings for at least three days. Our 'hit rate' for attacks is therefore over 50%.

Certain reservations have been expressed about the technique of ambulatory EEG monitoring: the limited scalp representation due to the limited number of channels, the difficulty in distinguishing artefact from genuine abnormality, and the possibility that some partial seizures may show no EEG change at the scalp.

Several authors have sought to elucidate these problems. Leroy and Ebersole (1983) reviewed a large number of EEG recordings and assessed the frequency with which interictal abnormalities occurred over different areas of the scalp. They then designed montages to record over the most likely areas and achieved a high success rate in the recording of interictal abnormalities, although their anteriorly based montages may require modification for use with children. Ebersole and Bridgers (1985) later showed that the limited number of EEG channels was not necessarily as great a disadvantage as previously thought. They recorded simultaneously three- and eight-channel ambulatory EEG and 16-channel cable telemetry using trifurcated electrodes. They showed that of 21 records regarded as epileptiform three-channel ambulatory recording detected and correctly lateralized 20 abnormalities and eight-channel detected 19. The false negative results consisted of interictal EEG abnormalities that were missed on review, a difficulty they note to be a particular problem with eight channels of information being replayed at such high speed. They found also that eight-channel recording, as would be expected, was far superior to three in showing the topographical distribution of abnormalities.

Although ambulatory recording can lateralize discharges no claims are made for the technique as a method of localizing epileptogenic foci. Not only does this require multi-channel recording but also depth recording and video techniques. However, Stores (1985) has shown that ambulatory monitoring and video recording are of equal value as aids to diagnosis. We have found it possible to video patients at the same time as ambulatory monitoring by synchronizing the video camera with the clock on the eight-channel recorder. Although this requires admission into hospital it still gives the patient some freedom. So far we have carried out the combined investigation on patients who have attacks in sleep and patients who are having very frequent attacks.

The problem of EEG artefact recognition has been discussed in detail by Blumhardt and Oozeer (1982). Familiarity with the artefacts produced by ambulant subjects can aid interpretation, as can the keeping of a diary sheet.

Muscle and movement artefacts inevitably occur at the time of attacks; in some the presence of postictal slowing is the only indication that seizures are genuine. In most partial attacks which we have recorded, the abnormality eventually becomes widespread and is discernible in areas not obscured by muscle activity. No conclusions can be made about attacks in which the EEG is totally obscured by artefact. Eight-channel recording is a great advantage in this respect. Of 86 attacks which we recorded on three channels 8% were not interpretable whereas of 29 attacks recorded on eight channels none was uninterpretable.

It is notable that even in some pseudoseizures a characteristic pattern is seen which consists of gross artefacts interspersed with periods of rest during which a normal alpha rhythm can be seen (Fig. 1). Perhaps the most pressing problem with ambulatory EEG recording is that some partial seizures, during which awareness is not impaired, may show no scalp EEG changes. Ives and Woods (1979) recorded 371 clinical and electrographical events on a four-channel ambulatory EEG recorder. No scalp changes were recorded for 21% of seizure events, and 58% of these consisted of simple partial attacks. In fact only 10% of simple partial seizures did show an EEG change. Before it can be assumed that attacks are not genuine, a description of the attack must be obtained to find out whether there really was any impairment of awareness.

In children, ambulatory monitoring is of particular value in the diagnosis and assessment of absence seizures. Parents and observers frequently underestimate the number of these attacks. The effect of absences on school performance, or in relation to specific events, can also be assessed. While absence seizures can be provoked in most patients by hyperventilation, this is not always so, and we found two of ten patients in whom spike and wave was seen in the 24-hour recording but not in the basic EEG.

Ambulatory monitoring can also be used for assessing the efficacy of anticonvulsant medication. Blomquist and Zetterlund (1985) evaluated the response to ethosuximide and Stefan *et al.* (1984) assessed once-daily administration of sodium valproate, using serial recordings to fine tune the dosage and establish the minimum effective daily dose. A similar study is being carried out in our own laboratory to assess the efficacy of once-daily vs twice-daily administration of sodium valproate. One such case is illustrated below.

CASE HISTORY

Martin was referred to the epilepsy clinic at the age of 20. He reported a history of blank spells beginning at 10 years of age which were manifested, among other things, as a tendency to switch off when being admonished and a habit of wandering off in the wrong direction when out shopping. An EEG recording at this time was abnormal, and a diagnosis of epilepsy was made. A range of anticonvulsants failed to have any appreciable effect, and this in turn exacerbated a tendency to poor compliance. Meanwhile, further EEGs up to the age of 18

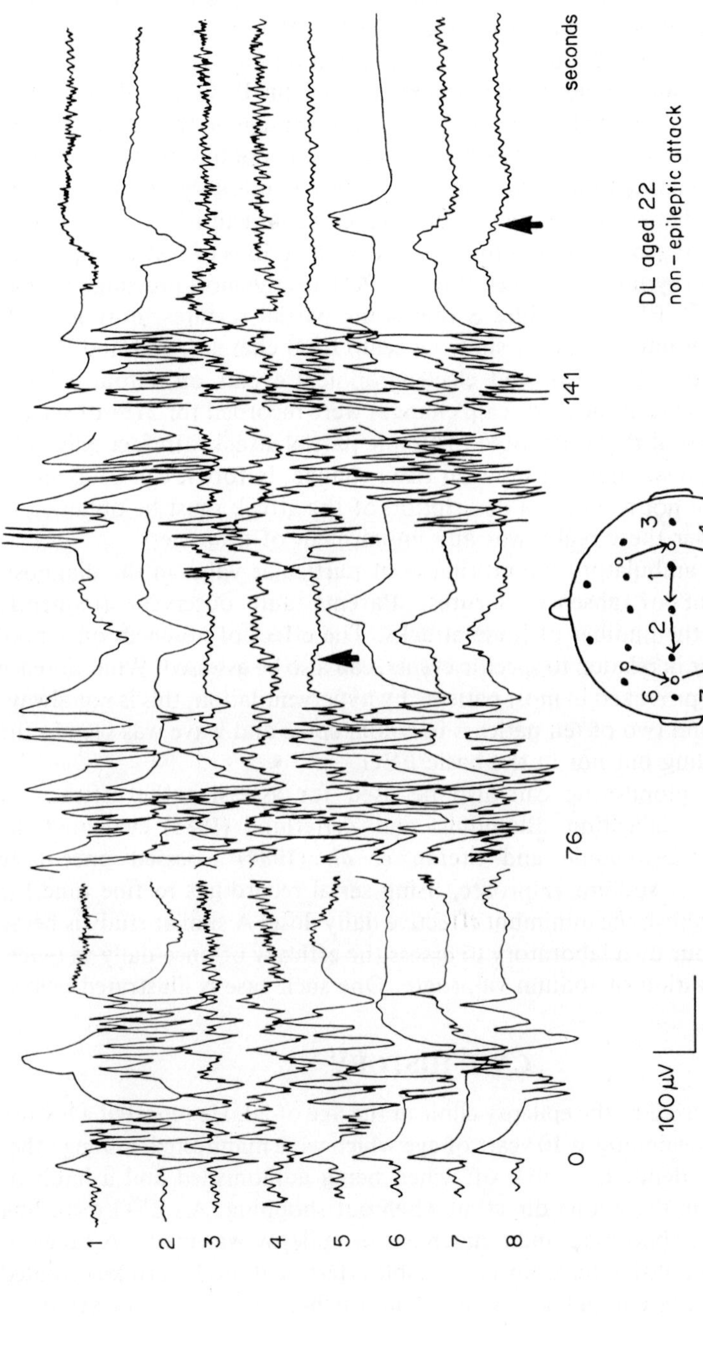

Fig. 1 Patient fell to ground and made sporadic jerking and thrashing movements. Arrows indicate 9–10 Hz alpha rhythm between bursts of artefact

years showed no abnormality. At 18 Martin was admitted to a local hospital for a week's assessment during which time he was told to keep a record of attacks. He was discharged from hospital still receiving medication but was told that his attacks might be of a psychological nature. At this point he totally refused to take further medication.

At the time of coming to the epilepsy clinic he was completing his college education and would soon be looking for work. His mother felt that his chances of gaining employment would be impaired by attacks occurring during interviews. Martin's main concern, however, was to acquire a driving licence. A basic EEG again showed no abnormality and so he was referred for ambulatory EEG recording.

During the application of electrodes several attacks were noted although there was no clinical signs other than a tendency to lose track of the conversation. When this was pointed out, he said he was often aware that he had missed something. A girlfriend who drove Martin to and from the clinic had at times observed some eyelid flutter and noted that occasionally she could abort attacks by waving her hand in front of his face.

During 24 hours of recording the EEG showed 197 discharges of 3–4 Hz spike and wave activity in waking, totalling 808 seconds. The mean duration was four seconds. Martin pressed the event button on six occasions during which spike and wave activity lasting between four and six seconds was observed.

He was then started on a single low dose of sodium valproate at night, and the recording was repeated. After a total of eight recordings and alterations in dosage and regimen we managed to reduce the number of discharges to five

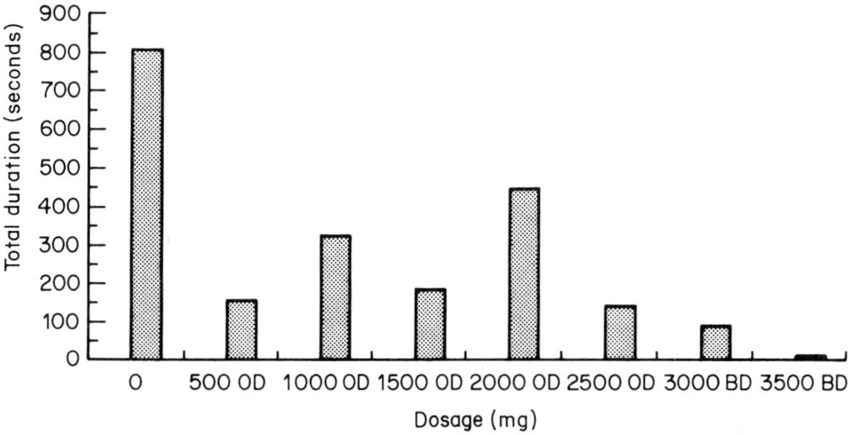

Fig. 2 Total duration of discharges during 24 hours' monitoring as an indicator of patient's response to treatment. Sodium valproate, given initially in a single dose at night and then changed to divided doses, achieved control at 38 mg/kg bodyweight

totalling 12 seconds (Fig. 2) with only the very occasional attack not on a recording day. After each recording Martin was informed of his progress. Knowledge of the reduction of discharges gave him the encouragement he needed to comply with his medication. The dosage is now 38 mg/kg bodyweight which we accept is rather high, although Martin himself would be happy to increase it in the hope of being able to obtain a driving licence in the future. He now has a permanent job which involves frequent contact with members of the public, a job which six months ago would have been out of the question.

Although this patient needed a high dose to control attacks, in other patients we have found discharges to be controlled at unexpectedly low doses, and ambulatory monitoring has enabled us to tune the dosage regimen very precisely.

Other reported applications of ambulatory monitoring have included the assessment of episodes of disturbed behaviour in children (Forrest and Crawford, 1981). Among the alternative diagnoses to epilepsy were: imaginary companion, habit spasm, and simulated seizures (which only occurred in children with a history of epilepsy).

Bachman (1984) also used ambulatory recording to diagnose 'spells' in two groups of children with and without a history of epilepsy. In three out of eight patients with a definite history of epilepsy the 'spell' proved to be a seizure whereas in only two of the 11 patients without a history of epilepsy was this the case.

Green *et al.* (1984) used combined EEG and ECG recording in 100 patients who were divided into three age groups. Their findings suggested that between birth and 20 years seizures were the most likely diagnosis whereas in those of 60 years and over, ECG abnormality was the most likely finding.

PRELIMINARY FOLLOW-UP STUDY

To look for any differences between children and adults we reviewed our own first 215 recordings. One hundred and seven patients (just over half of them children) experienced attacks which were interpretable. If we assume that a negative EEG finding makes a diagnosis of epilepsy unlikely then there seems to be an equal likelihood in children that attacks will be epileptic or non-epileptic, with 50% showing no EEG abnormality. Thus unexplained attacks in children referred for ambulatory monitoring produce positive evidence for epilepsy in about half the cases. In adults, however, attacks are more likely to be accompanied by negative EEG findings (78%), making a diagnosis of epilepsy unlikely (Table 1). The kind of attacks which occurred during recording are shown in Table 2. In adults the most common attacks were partial seizures with a right-sided predominance. In children, as would be expected, absence seizures were almost as frequent a finding as partial seizures. A number of attacks remained unclassified because there was no clinical observation of them or the EEG changes were too complex to be categorized using a three-channel recorder.

Table 1. EEG findings during attacks in 61 children and 46 adults

Age (years)	EEG Abnormal	EEG No abnormality
Under 21	30	31
21 and over	10	36
Combined	40	67

Table 2. Types of epileptic seizure recorded in 30 children and ten adults

Attacks	Age (years) Under 21	Age (years) 21 and over
Absence	9	1
Tonic-clonic	2	1
Myoclonic	1	1
Right partial	9	5
Left partial	3	1
Unclassified	6	1

In a more detailed study of the children whose attacks were unaccompanied by EEG abnormality, they were classified according to their anticonvulsant medication at the time of investigation (Table 3). Results showed that half of the children were receiving such drugs and half were not. Almost a quarter of the patients were receiving two drugs; one of these had a definite history of epilepsy as well as episodic symptoms of an uncertain nature. One other patient who was receiving one drug also had a definite history of epilepsy as well as the attacks under investigation. Thus, of the 15 patients receiving medication, two were being treated for an additional definite seizure disorder.

All patients receiving medication at the time of the recording were followed up. The referring specialists were asked whether, at the last consultation, the patient was still receiving medication, whether attacks were still occurring, and the final diagnosis (Table 4). The results showed that six patients were no longer receiving antiepileptic drugs and in five, attacks had ceased. Four of these were

Table 3. Medication being taken at the time of recording by 31 patients under the age of 21 years. Bracketed numbers indicate patients with definite epileptic seizures in addition to the attacks under investigation

Antiepileptic drugs	Patients
None	16
One	4 (1)
Two	7 (1)
One + benzodiazepine	3
Benzodiazepine alone	1

Table 4. Results of follow-up in patients under 21 years who were receiving medication at the time of recording but whose EEG showed no abnormality during attacks

Patient	Antiepileptic drugs	Attacks	Final diagnosis	Follow-up (months)
1	–	–	Reaction to events	22
2	–	–	Emotional	60
3	–	–	Night terrors	14
4	–	–	Developed schizophrenia	57
5	–	–	Emotional	19
6	–	?	Psychological	12
7	+	+	Epilepsy	48
8*	+	+	Partial seizures	16
9	+	+	Epilepsy	24
10	+	–	Epilepsy	42
11†	+	–	Panic	22
12†	+	+	Psychological	24

*Clinical description of attack implied no loss of awareness.
†Definite history of epilepsy plus episodic symptoms of uncertain nature.

thought to be suffering from an emotional disturbance; there was one case of night terrors and one patient developed schizophrenia.

In four patients the final diagnosis was epilepsy and three of these were still receiving antiepileptic drugs and also experiencing attacks. As our results had shown that attacks in these patients were not associated with EEG abnormality, we reviewed them in more detail. In one we found that during the recorded attack there was no loss of awareness, so it was possible that there had been no scalp EEG changes. In two the current attacks differ clinically from those which we had recorded, and in the fourth, attacks had ceased while on medication and were assumed to be due to epilepsy.

Of the two patients who had a definite history of epilepsy as well as the episodic symptoms under investigation, the episodic symptoms ceased in one but in both the attacks were regarded as non-epileptic. Two patients were lost to follow up.

We feel that in such a select group of patients being treated with antiepileptic drugs these results are encouraging. Obviously further work is required to follow up patients who were not receiving medication and also those in whom abnormality was found at the time of attacks.

REFERENCES

Bachman, D. S. (1984) 24-hour ambulatory electroencephalographic monitoring in pediatrics. *Clin. Electroencephalogr.*, **15**, 164–166.

Blomquist, H. and Zetterlund, B. (1985) Evaluation of treatment in typical absence seizures. *Acta Paediatr. Scand.*, **74**, 409–415.

BLUMHARDT, L. D. and OOZEER, R. (1982) Problems encountered in the interpretation of ambulatory EEG recordings. In: *Mobile Long-term EEG Monitoring*, H. Stefan and W. Burr (Eds), Gustav Fischer, Stuttgart, New York, pp. 37–50.

EBERSOLE, J. S. and BRIDGERS, S. L. (1985) Direct comparison of three- and eight-channel ambulatory cassette EEG with intensive inpatient monitoring. *Neurology*, **35**, 846–854.

FORREST, G. C. and CRAWFORD, C. (1981) Ambulatory monitoring and child psychiatry. In: *Papers on Electroencephalography ISAM, Ghent*, F. D. Stott *et al.* (Eds), Academic Press, London, pp. 157–161.

GREEN, J., SCALES, D., NEALIS, J. and KING, A. (1984) Further experience with ambulatory EEG monitoring. *J. Fla. Med. Assoc.*, **71**, 17–20.

IVES, J. R. and WOODS, J. F. (1979) A study of 100 patients with focal epilepsy using a four-channel ambulatory cassette recorder. In: *Proceedings of the Third International Symposium on Ambulatory Monitoring*, F. D. Stott *et al.* (Eds), Academic Press, London, pp. 383–392.

LEROY, R. F. and EBERSOLE, J. S. (1983) An evaluation of ambulatory EEG monitoring: montage design. *Neurology*, **33**, 1–7.

STEFAN, H., BURR, W., FISCHEL, H., FROSCHER, W. and PENIN, H. (1984) Intensive follow-up monitoring in patients with once-daily evening administration of sodium valproate. *Epilepsia*, **25**, 152–160.

STORES, G. (1985) Comparison of video and ambulatory (cassette) monitoring in the investigation of attacks in children. In: *Proceedings of the Fifth International Symposium on Ambulatory Monitoring, Padua*, C. Dal Palu and A. C. Pessina (Eds), Cleup, Padova, pp. 633–638.

DISCUSSION

Dr C. M. Verity (Cambridge): You say that some partial seizures may not be accompanied by EEG changes in the scalp. Do you mean that there is no scalp change or that it cannot be picked up by ambulatory monitoring?

Powell: These are seizures that consist only of an aura and quite often show no scalp EEG changes even on a 16-channel EEG.

Professor C. R. B. Joyce (Switzerland): Your eight-channel recorder looks fine for girls with long hair, but what about the other girls and the boys?

Powell: The amplifiers can be concealed beneath the hair, even if it is quite short. A scarf around the neck or turning the collar up conceals the leads quite well, and we have patients who go to school or work quite happily.

Verity: Sometimes part of the clinical picture is difficult behaviour, and the neurologists may be reluctant to allow their precious equipment to be put at risk. Is that a practical problem in your experience?

Powell: At first we did insist that difficult patients should be kept in hospital for the duration of the recording. In practice, the nurses were so busy that they could not supervise the patients all day, and we achieved more success by letting the patients go home. The mother would be far more watchful.

Epilepsy in Young People
Edited by E. Ross, D. Chadwick and R. Crawford

15

New techniques in investigation

J. STEPHENSON
Royal Hospital for Sick Children, Glasgow

SUMMARY

Several new techniques are contributing to the investigation of epilepsy. One of the simplest ways of describing a seizure precisely is to make a video recording. With other methods, this has considerably improved understanding of epileptic falls in relation to axial spasm and infantile spasm. New biochemical monitoring procedures likely to contribute to the field of epilepsy include CSF amino acid analysis, neurotransmitter and neuromodulator detection, and mass spectroscopy of organic derivatives.

Of the techniques used to display focal abnormalities in localized areas of the brain, perhaps computerized ultrasound has the most value in the very young infant. X-ray computerized tomography (CT) scanning, magnetic resonance imaging (MRI), positron emission tomography (PET) scanning and single photon emission computerized tomography (SPECT) each have advantages in picking out some aetiologies of focal epilepsy. Dipole localization method (DLM) has potential for identifying deep intracranial foci. However, in practice, depth electrode studies are the final arbiters of localization when epilepsy surgery is planned.

The new techniques now being applied to investigation of epilepsy fall under three main headings:

1. Improving the definition and *description of the seizure* itself in clinical and neurophysiological terms.
2. Investigation into the *biochemical mechanisms* of seizures, particularly in the neonatal period.
3. *Neuro-imaging*, as an aid to lesional and genetic diagnosis, and before neurosurgery.

These three categories overlap to some extent but provide a framework for critical discussion of techniques which range from the fairly simple to the extremely complex and expensive.

SEIZURE DESCRIPTION

Accurate description of epilepsy is an absolute prerequisite for its investigation (Gilchrist, 1985; Kiok *et al.*, 1986). Video recording of seizures is one of the simplest ways of improving and refining the description of a seizure, as demonstrated by a recent study on the lateralizing significance of versive head and eye movements (Wyllie *et al.*, 1986). A blind assessment of head and eye movements, captured by high quality video recordings, was compared with EEG evidence of the side of origin of the habitual epileptic seizures in these patients.

Defining versive movements as clonic or tonic head and eye deviations—unquestionably forced and involuntary—resulting in sustained and unnatural positioning of the head and eyes as demonstrated on the videotape, Wyllie *et al.* found that versive eye movements were always directed contralaterally to the electrical origin of the seizures. By contrast, non-versive lateral head and eye movements occurred equally away from and towards the electrical site of seizure origin. This videotape study also showed that seizures arising from areas outside the temporal lobe usually began with contraversion whereas in seizures of temporal lobe origin the versive head movement was always preceded by quiet staring or staring with automatisms. Indeed, when contraversion was preceded by staring with automatisms the seizures were always of temporal origin.

For comparatively simple and inexpensive simultaneous video recording, the method used by Dr James Manson in Adelaide Children's Hospital deserves wider use. He employs a video camera in the EEG department which records continuously throughout the working day. A real-time display in seconds is also recorded continuously both on the videotape and on the EEG paper. If any seizure occurs spontaneously or is induced by some manoeuvre, then that part of the video recording is retained and can be compared with the standard EEG recordings using real time.

Considerably more expensive in terms of resources are the methods of so-called intensive monitoring using video-EEG with either cable or radiotelemetry. Two general methods are in use. One is to make a simultaneous video and EEG display which can be replayed on split-screen or other superimposed system in slow motion, and to undertake separate high quality polygraphic studies of the seizure by means of surface electromyography (EMG) and other procedures (Egli *et al.*, 1985). The other method involves transmitting and simultaneously displaying the EEG and polygraphic material such as surface EMG and once again replaying this material on the video recorder in slow motion (Ikeno *et al.*, 1985). As an example, both these methods have substantially improved our understanding of the mechanisms of epileptic falls such as those seen in the so-called Lennox–Gastaut syndrome.

Previously terms such as akinetic, myoclonic and atonic were used loosely and often incorrectly to describe the falls in any given child. From these new intensive monitoring studies it has become clear that one of the most common seizure types coinciding with a fall in early life is the axial spasm well known to paediatricians as the infantile spasm. Other seizure types manifesting as falls include tonic, myoclonic-atonic and atonic seizures, with various additional combinations of seizures occurring both before and after the ictal event responsible for the fall.

It seems likely that in much the same way that once phonocardiography had refined the classification of various heart sounds and murmurs so that thereafter sophisticated cardiac diagnosis was possible by using the stethoscope alone, so once a sufficient body of knowledge has been obtained by intensive video EEG monitoring it should become possible to diagnose these various epileptic falls by less elaborate methods, perhaps by observation alone. Considerable problems, however, remain to be solved with respect to the analysis of limbic seizures.

BIOCHEMICAL MECHANISMS

New techniques seem likely to contribute to understanding of the epilepsies, but are of very limited practical value at present. For example, amino acid analysis of the cerebrospinal fluid is helpful in the diagnosis of glycine encephalopathy as a cause of severe myoclonic epilepsy of the neonate, but of little else.

Techniques of organic acid analysis have improved, moving from gas liquid chromatography (GLC) via mass spectroscopy (GLC-MS) to fast atom bombardment (FAB-MS). Once again, although there is a suggestion, for example, that some cases of MCT acyl co-enzyme A dehydrogenase deficiency present as a seizure disorder, the epidemiology and veracity of such observations is still obscure. Comprehensive biochemical studies are rarely performed on children with epilepsy, and it is not possible to judge the general incidence of such findings as a disorder of purine metabolism (Coleman *et al.*, 1986).

It is also possible to measure various neurotransmitters and neuromodulator molecules in the cerebrospinal fluid, such as GABA and the biogenic amines and their metabolites, but as yet these investigations have no firm place in epilepsy investigations.

NEURO-IMAGING

Use of techniques to display focal abnormalities in localized areas of the brain has been largely determined by the availability of neurosurgical treatment for focal epilepsies. However, recognition of anatomical abnormalities and particularly those due to genetic disorders can also improve management. Tuberous sclerosis is the most common disorder that can be displayed by imaging studies, even when cutaneous signs are minimal, although the gene defect may be present despite comprehensive negative investigations.

Among anatomical imaging techniques, computerized ultrasound may be of the most value in the very young infant, though few data are so far available.

Thanks to progressive advances, X-ray CT scanning can now reveal smaller lesions which may be associated with focal epilepsies, but the effect this will have on management has not yet been clearly described. The use of iodide contrast in the CSF to clarify the anatomy of the mesial temporal structures has also been advocated.

Magnetic resonance imaging (Lesser *et al.*, 1986; Mazziotta and Engel, 1985; McLachlan *et al.*, 1985) has the potential to reveal more of the cerebral malformations responsible for some types of refractory focal epilepsy. In one recent study (McLachlan *et al.*, 1985) three out of ten patients with intractable focal seizures exhibited areas of increased signal density on T_2-weighted images in the mesial portion of the temporal lobe, from which the seizures were shown to arise, without obvious changes on CT scan.

Positron emission tomography (PET) scanning (Engel, 1985; Mazziotta and Engel, 1985) remains too expensive for widespread use. It has shown localized raised metabolism during seizures and focal low metabolism in interictal periods. A more generally accessible method is single-photon emission computerized tomography (SPECT) (Mazziotta and Engel, 1985), which seems likely to become an essential preliminary to epilepsy surgery.

This brief review can only touch on new techniques of what may be called EEG imaging, but the practical value of 'brain mapping' has yet to be demonstrated. So-called 'stereo electroencephalography' using multiple depth electrodes is an invasive technique regarded by some as an essential prerequisite for epilepsy surgery. An entirely non-invasive and potentially valuable method for localizing deep intracranial sources of the EEG has recently been published using a computer assisted mathematical model based on electrical field theory (Smith *et al.*, 1986). This technique, the so-called dipole localization method (DLM), has been found to localize induced electrical discharges reliably. Finally, magnetoencephalography is a promising method for demonstrating the localization of abnormal neural activity through endogenous alteration of the magnetic field, but its clinical usefulness has yet to be demonstrated.

CONCLUSION

Despite the increasing array of techniques the choice and value of such investigations in a child with epilepsy remain limited. However, the assessment of any new form of therapy, whether surgical or medical, demands the most exact description of the epilepsy that techniques allow.

REFERENCES

COLEMAN, M., LANDGREBE, M. and LANDGREBE, A. (1986) Purine seizure disorders. *Epilepsia*, **27**, 263–269.

EGLI, M., MOTHERSILL, I., O'KANE, M. and O'KANE, F. (1985) The axial spasm—the predominant type of drop seizure in patients with secondary generalised epilepsy. *Epilepsia*, **26**, 401–415.

ENGEL, J. (1985) Positron emission tomography (PET) in the diagnosis of epilepsy. In: *The Epilepsies*, R. J. Porter and P. L. Morselli (Eds), Butterworth, London, p. 242.

GILCHRIST, J. M. (1985) Arrhythmogenic seizures: diagnosis by simultaneous EEG/ECG recording. *Neurology*, **35**, 1503–1506.

IKENO, T., SHIGEMATSU, H., MIYAKOSHI, M., OHBA, A., YAGI, K. and SEINO, M. (1985) An analytic study of epileptic falls. *Epilepsia*, **26**, 612–621.

KIOK, M. C., TERRENCE, C. F., FROMM, G. H. and LAVINE, S. (1986) Sinus arrest in epilepsy. *Neurology*, **36**, 115–116.

LESSER, R. P., MODIC, M. T., WEINSTEIN, M. A., DUCHESNEAN, P. M., LÜDERS, H., DINNER, D. S., MORRIS, H. H., ESTES, M., CHOU, S. M. and HAHN, J. F. (1986) Magnetic resonance imaging (1.5 Tesla) in patients with intractable focal seizures. *Arch. Neurol.*, **43**, 367–371.

MAZZIOTTA, J. C. and ENGEL, J. (1985) Advanced neuro-imaging techniques in the study of human epilepsy: PET, SPECT, and NMR-CT. In: *Recent Advances in Epilepsy 2*, T. A. Pedley and B. S. Meldrum (Eds), Churchill Livingstone, Edinburgh, p. 65.

MCLACHLAN, R. S., NICHOLSON, R. L., BLACK, S., CARR, T. and BLUME, W. T. (1985) Nuclear magnetic resonance imaging, a new approach to the investigation of refractory temporal lobe epilepsy. *Epilepsia*, **26**, 555–562.

SMITH, D. B., SIDMAN, R. D., FLANIGAN, H., HENKE, J. and LABINER, D. (1986) Available method for localising deep intracranial sources of the EEG. *Neurology*, **35**, 1702–1707.

WYLLIE, E., LÜDERS, H., MORRIS, H. H., LESSER, R. P. and DINNER, D. S. (1986) The lateralising significance of versive head and eye movements during epileptic seizures. *Neurology*, **36**, 606–611.

DISCUSSION

Dr D. L. Stevens (Gloucester): You only touched briefly on electrical methods of brain mapping. Can you say whether these new techniques really serve a useful purpose or whether they are yet another example of a technical trick that doesn't necessarily serve as a method of clinical investigation?

Stephenson: We have had two varieties in our department and used them on patients without being convinced of their clinical value. But this might be a fault in me . . . .

Dr M. R. Trimble (London), Chairman: Positron emission tomography (PET) has contributed a great deal to our knowledge of the interictal state of patients with epilepsy, but its clinical value is at present largely confined to investigation of patients with focal seizures awaiting surgery. Glucose PET has been found useful by the UCLA group in the assessment of their cases. It may eventually replace intracerebral electrodes for gathering information about the site of an epileptic focus. With regard to magnetic resonance imaging (MRI), we have just completed scanning 50 cases, and have picked up one lesion which has altered our diagnosis and treatment, compared with what we already knew from CT scanning. Recent American experience suggests that the pick-up rate for tumours in new referrals—which our cases were not—is increased by using MRI.

Epilepsy in Young People
Edited by E. Ross, D. Chadwick and R. Crawford

16

Photosensitive epilepsy and visual display units

ARNOLD J. WILKINS
MRC Applied Psychology Unit, Cambridge

SUMMARY

About 4% of patients with epilepsy are liable to visually-induced seizures. A variety of visual stimuli can be responsible, ranging from flickering sunlight and striped shirts to intermittent cathode-ray tube displays such as television. The epileptogenic properties of intermittent cathode-ray tube displays are related to:

1. The size of the screen and the distance from which it is viewed, which together determine: (a) the area of retina stimulated, and (b) whether any line pattern from the raster will be of the critical retinal size. Screens with 312 lines should be viewed from a distance that is at least four times the width of the screen.
2. The frequency with which the screen is 'refreshed'. Many patients are sensitive at 50 per second, very few at 60 per second and above.
3. The presence of line interlace. This doubles the number of lines and effectively halves the refresh rate. If the screen is large enough and is viewed from a short distance the interlacing lines can form a highly epileptogenic pattern.
4. The nature of the material displayed. (Flashing graphics are best avoided; closely-spaced text can be mildly epileptogenic.)
5. The room illumination: dim lighting may be preferable.

The nature of individual sensitivity also has to be considered in advising photosensitive patients.

INTRODUCTION

Many general statements from a wide variety of sources have sought to reassure the public about the use of visual display units. For example, it has been claimed that the risk of a seizure is slight and that a VDU will never induce a photosensitive seizure unless the individual has already had seizures under other circumstances. These reassurances are too general. They do not do justice to the complexity of the issues involved which derive firstly from the way in which photosensitivity varies from patient to patient, and secondly from the enormous range of displays. VDUs vary so widely that it is impossible to talk about the risk that their use involves without specifying their characteristics. In short, some VDUs are most unlikely to produce a seizure in any photosensitive patient, while others are quite likely to do so in certain cases.

To determine whether a patient is likely to be sensitive to a display, a knowledge of the spatial and temporal characteristics of the display needs to be combined with information about the spatial and temporal characteristics of the patient's sensitivity, derived mainly from EEG studies.

About 4% of patients with epilepsy are liable to visually-induced seizures. The majority of these patients, and a few others besides, demonstrate a photoconvulsive EEG response to intermittent photic stimulation. The characteristics of this response have been described elsewhere (Newmark and Penry, 1979, Chapter 5): this study concentrates on the stimulus characteristics that bring about such a response. It is from studies of these characteristics that we can predict the type of VDU that is likely to present a problem.

CHARACTERISTICS OF VISUAL DISPLAY UNITS

Certain very broad generalizations can be made. The large majority of VDUs use a cathode ray tube. In the cathode ray tube a beam of electrons is projected on to the phosphor coating of the screen where it creates a bright spot of light. Usually the beam scans the whole screen systematically, starting at the top of the screen and tracing a series of closely spaced horizontal lines. The intensity of the beam and thus the brightness of the spot is varied electronically as it scans down the screen so as to produce the desired pattern of light and dark. This form of scan is known as a raster. The frequency with which the beam scans from the top to the bottom of the screen (the refresh rate) varies considerably from one VDU to another but is generally within the range 50–100 per second.

The majority of VDUs used in schools resemble domestic television in that the scan rate is 50/second. In the series of susceptible patients studied by Jeavons and Harding (1975) nearly 50% exhibited a photoconvulsive response in the EEG when exposed to diffuse intermittent light with a frequency of 50/second. It has been argued that this figure may be unrepresentative because their series included many patients with television-induced epilepsy. Representative or not, it remains the case that photosensitive patients can be sensitive to flicker at a frequency of 50/second. It is much less common, however, for patients to be sensitive when the frequency is 60/second (Jeavons and Harding, 1975). Many office VDUs now have refresh rates of 60/second and above.

Fig. 1 An epileptogenic pattern. The stripes have equal width and spacing and have a high contrast. At a viewing distance of 40 cm each stripe subtends about 10 minutes of arc at the eye

The number of lines in the raster scan varies from display to display, although the minimum is usually 312. The number of lines is critical because the effects of flicker can be exacerbated by pattern. Some patterns are far worse than others, striped patterns being particularly bad (Fig. 1). Epileptiform EEG abnormalities are most likely when each strip subtends about 10 minutes of arc at the eye (Wilkins *et al.*, 1980). The angle subtended by the stripes from a raster scan is determined by the number of lines, the size of the screen and the distance from which is it viewed. If there are 312 lines on a screen with a diagonal measurement of 26 inches (660 mm), each line subtends 10 minutes of arc when the viewing distance is 18 inches (450 mm). When the entire screen is lit it therefore has spatial characteristics close to those that are maximally provocative. As the viewing distance increases and the retinal image of the lines gets smaller, the epileptogenic effect decreases. When the lines subtend less than about four minutes of arc their effect can be ignored. On a 26 inch (660 mm) screen with 312 lines, each line subtends four minutes of arc at a viewing distance of six feet (1.8 m). Screens rarely have fewer than 312 lines, so a useful rule of thumb is that the effects of the raster pattern can be ignored when the viewing distance is more than four times the width of the screen.

Sometimes the scan is interlaced, that is to say, on one scan from the top to the bottom of the screen odd numbered lines appear, and on the next even numbered lines. The odd and even scans alternate continuously, creating stripes that are refreshed at half the scan frequency. Interlace is used when fine detail is required since twice as many lines can be displayed for a given scan rate without visible flicker. When the scan rate is 50/second, as it is on most VDUs used in schools, each line appears 25 times per second, and the pattern the lines create is similar to a pattern of stripes that repeatedly change phase (white-black; black-white) at this frequency. A pattern of stripes that reverses in phase in this way can be far more epileptogenic than a stable pattern, particularly when the frequency of reversal is close to 20/second. Over 70% of photosensitive patients are sensitive to patterns of stripes of this kind.

Whether or not the display interlaces depends on certain characteristics of the video signal, and in the majority of schools' computers these characteristics are under software control from the computer. On the BBC micro, for example, the interlace can be suppressed in all modes except mode 7 by typing *TVO,1 before changing mode.

When a VDU screen is less than 25 cm (12 inches) in diagonal measurement the stripes from the conventional 312-line raster scan play little or no part in epileptogenesis, regardless of the viewing distance (Wilkins *et al.*, 1979). This is presumably because the viewing distances which would be close enough to provide a sufficiently large retinal image of the lines to induce epilepsy are too close for accommodation to be maintained, and the image of the lines is poorly focused. As a result, the presence or absence of line interlace is less important for small screens. Sometimes, however, the interlace can affect the edge of contours in the image drawn on the screen, producing visible flicker.

Provided the brightness is taken into account, the colour of intermittent light does not affect its epileptogenic properties, with the exception that deep red light may be more epileptogenic (Binnie *et al.*, 1984) and blue light slightly less so (Jeavons and Harding, 1975). The likelihood with which epileptiform EEG abnormalities are induced by monochrome and colour televisions does not differ significantly (Wilkins *et al.*, 1979) and so it would appear unlikely that the colour of a display, as such, has much effect on the likelihood of epileptiform EEG abnormalities. However, the colour of the light emitted by a VDU is determined by the phosphor, and phosphors differ in their persistence, i.e. the extent to which light continues to be emitted after excitation by the electron beam has ceased. Slow phosphors which emit light for a long time are used on some textual displays to provide a flicker-free image when the refresh rate is low. Although such displays may be comfortable to look at, their use is not widespread because they have the disadvantage that when the display is changed, 'ghosts' of the previous display remain for a while. 'Fast' phosphors are more commonly used, particularly for graphics. The persistence of the phosphor determines the depth of modulation of the intermittent light from the display. There is only very little information on the depth of temporal modulation of light necessary for epileptogenesis. The data are confined to recordings from one patient who viewed sinusoidally modulated diffuse light at a variety of modulation depths. Modulation of as little as 10% was sufficient to induce epileptiform EEG abnormalities (Wilkins and Lindsay, 1985). The depth of modulation from VDUs is usually greatly in excess of this figure.

OTHER INFLUENCES ON PHOTOSENSITIVITY

The nature of the material displayed on the screen is as important as the display itself. If little of the screen is lit, intermittent light can have little effect. The greater the illuminated area, the greater its effects, and for this reason bright text on a dark background may be preferable to the reverse contrast. If flashing graphics are displayed, as is the case in many computer games, the effects of the intermittent refresh may be compounded. There are also other, more subtle, sources of potentially epileptogenic stimulation. These have to do with the spatial properties of text. The successive lines of text can provide a pattern of stripes with characteristics within the epileptogenic range. Stripes are more likely to induce seizures when they have even width and spacing (Wilkins *et al.*, 1984), so it is important for text to be double spaced.

The room illumination can also be relevant. Binnie *et al.* (1980a) noted that patients who were sensitive to television only at close viewing distances (that is, not sensitive at frequencies of 50 per second) were more likely to exhibit epileptiform EEG abnormalities when the room lights were turned on.

There are many other aspects of displays that may be important, but I have restricted discussion to those about which we have data concerning photosensitivity.

Sensitivity to both intermittent light and patterns is usually considerably reduced, if not eliminated, by covering one eye. If the light is intermittent it is necessary to cover the orbit to prevent light reaching the retina through the closed eyelid. A cosmetic and selective way of occluding one eye when using a VDU is to provide the patient with a pair of glasses, one lens of which is polarized at an angle of 90 degrees to the axis of polarization of a sheet of polarizer placed in front of the VDU screen. This method is more acceptable than an eye patch and can be useful when conventional therapy is ineffective or inappropriate (Wilkins and Lindsay, 1985).

The stimuli which provoke seizures in photosensitive patients may provoke feelings of visual discomfort in others. The above remarks may therefore be taken to apply with equal force to discomfort experienced by visual display unit operators (Wilkins *et al.*, 1984). This is not to imply that the epileptogenic properties of displays provide the only source of 'eye-strain': the intermittent light can affect ocular motor control and this may also be responsible for discomfort (Wilkins, 1986).

INDIVIDUAL DIFFERENCES

The above remarks apply to photosensitivity in general. There are, however, important differences in the sensitivity of individual patients. The variation in the frequency range of sensitivity to intermittent light has already been touched on, but there are many other differences. Perhaps one of the most dramatic is the area of retinal stimulation necessary for epileptogenesis: some patients are sensitive to very small patterns of stripes, others are sensitive only when the pattern size becomes very large. Some patients are sensitive to stripes only when they have a limited range of orientation, and this orientation selectivity can appear independently of any astigmatism (Wilkins *et al.*, 1980).

A substantial proportion of patients, perhaps as many as 20%, appear to self-induce seizures; they exhibit a slow upward movement of the eyelids that is often accompanied by paroxysmal EEG activity (Binnie *et al.*, 1980b; Wastell *et al.*, 1982). A few patients use the television to induce seizures, and will deliberately seek out opportunties to get close to it; in others the attraction to the set appears to be less an act of will than a capture of the will by subclinical seizure activity. These patients have a compulsive attraction to the set, approach it in a daze, and gaze at the screen, often with their noses touching it. The polarized monocular occlusion mentioned above can be an effective treatment (Wilkins and Lindsay, 1985), but monocular occlusion does not reduce light sensitivity in all patients (Jeavons and Harding, 1975).

Some idea of the likely sensitivity of individual patients to VDUs can be determined from the EEG examination. If the EEG exhibits a 'photoconvulsive' response to light with a frequency close to 50 flashes per second, the patient is likely to be at risk from a conventional television at normal viewing distances, and also from a VDU that has a 50/second refresh rate. If, as is more common, the patient is sensitive only to lower frequency light, then the risk from television and VDUs should be considerably less. Nevertheless, if any EEG photosensitivity is demonstrated it is a wise precaution for a patient to avoid close exposure to a large screen, particularly if it has a 25/second interlace. During the EEG examination it is useful to check whether covering one eye protects the patient from the effects of intermittent light, and if so, which eye is more effective.

The routine EEG examination does not usually include assessment of pattern sensitivity. Although the majority of pattern-sensitive patients are also sensitive to intermittent diffuse light (as used in the conventional EEG examination), the presence of pattern sensitivity cannot be predicted from the response to intermittent light, and has therefore to be assessed separately. About 30% of patients who are sensitive to intermittent light are sensitive also to static continuously-illuminated patterns of stripes, provided the stripes have the maximal provocative stimulus characteristics. As already mentioned, when the stripes vibrate or change phase at roughly 20 cycles/second, about 70% of patients are sensitive. Ascertaining the presence of pattern sensitivity can help distinguish the patients who are likely to be sensitive to the raster scan (Stefansson *et al.*, 1977), and if pattern sensitivity is very pronounced it can provide an indication that the patient is likely to be sensitive to the striped characteristics of textual displays. If seizures are provoked by reading, they can sometimes be prevented by covering the lines of text above and below those being read using a simple mask (the Cambridge Easy Reader*).

Of course, the EEG findings can give no more than an indication of patients' sensitivity at the time of recording, and such sensitivity can vary considerably from day to day. The findings therefore provide only a rough guide and need to be interpreted in the light of the history. When taking a history it is important to remember that seizures may take the form of a fleeting impairment of cognitive function (Aarts *et al.*, 1984) and can therefore pass unnoticed, particularly if a patient is engrossed with a computer.

ADVICE FOR PHOTOSENSITIVE PATIENTS

Notwithstanding the differences between patients, the following advice will be appropriate for the majority of sufferers:

If at all possible, use a VDU with a refresh rate of 60/second or above.
The VDU should have a small screen (less than about 0.25m (12 inches)).
Avoid exposure to large VDU screens with a 50/second refresh rate, particularly those with a 25/second interlace.
Conventional televisions with a large screen should not be used as a VDU. If it is necessary to use a large screen it is essential that the line interlace be switched off.

Further guidance for patients and families is given by the questions and answers that follow this contribution.

*Obtainable from Engineering and Design Plastics, 84 High Street, Cherry Hinton, Cambridge CB1 4HZ, UK.

CAVEAT

This article has emphasized the characteristics of displays that may, under certain unusual circumstances, be responsible for the visual induction of seizures. The information should not be taken as indicating that there is a high risk of seizures associated with the use of visual display units. The degree of risk is extremely small, even in patients who are highly photosensitive. People with epilepsy already experience considerable difficulty obtaining employment, and their difficulty should not be permitted to increase simply because any employment would involve the use of visual display units. Very few patients with epilepsy are photosensitive, and, as has been shown, it is possible to minimize the chances of a seizure with the appropriate choice of display even in patients who are highly photosensitive.

REFERENCES

AARTS, J. H. P., BINNIE, C. D., SMIT, A. M. and WILKINS, A. J. (1984) Selective cognitive impairment during focal and generalised epileptiform EEG activity. *Brain*, **107**, 293–308.

BINNIE, C. D., DARBY, C. E., DE KORTE, R. A., VELDHUIZEN, R. and WILKINS, A. J. (1980a) EEG sensitivity to television: effects of ambient lighting. *Electroencephalogr. Clin. Neurophysiol.*, **50**, 329–331.

BINNIE, C. D., DARBY, C. E., DE KORTE, R. A. and WILKINS, A. J. (1980b) Self-induction of epileptic seizures by eye closure: incidence and recognition. *J. Neurol. Neurosurg. Psychiatry*, **43**, 386–389.

BINNIE C. D., ESTEVEZ, O., KASTELEIJN-NOLST TRENITE, D. G. A. and PETERS, A. (1984) Colour and photosensitive epilepsy. *Electroencephalogr. Clin. Neurophysiol.*, **58**, 387–391.

JEAVONS, P. M. and HARDING, G. F. A. (1975) *Photosensitive Epilepsy: a Review of the Literature and Study of 460 Patients*, Heinemann, London.

NEWMARK, M. E. and PENRY, J. K. (1979) *Photosensitivity and Epilepsy: a Review*, Raven Press, New York.

STEFANSSON, S. B., DARBY, C. E., WILKINS, A. J., BINNIE, C. D., MARLTON, A. P., SMITH, A. T. and STOCKLEY, A. V. (1977) Television epilepsy and pattern sensitivity. *Br. Med. J.*, **2**, 88–89.

WASTELL, D. G., WILKINS, A. J. and DARBY, C. E. (1982) Self-induction of epileptic seizures by eye closure: spectral analysis of concomitant EEG. *J. Neurol. Neurosurg. Psychiatry*, **45**, 1151–1152.

WILKINS, A. J. (1986) Intermittent illumination from visual display units and fluorescent lighting affects movement of eyes across text. *Human Factors*, **28**, 75–81.

WILKINS, A. J. and LINDSAY, J. (1985) Common forms of reflex epilepsy: physiological mechanisms and techniques for treatment. In: *Recent Advances in Epilepsy 2*, T. A. Pedley and B. S. Meldrum (Eds), Churchill Livingstone, Edinburgh, pp. 239–271.

WILKINS, A. J., DARBY, C. E., BINNIE, C. D., STEFANSSON, S. F., JEAVONS, P. M. and HARDING, G. F. A. (1979) Television epilepsy—the role of pattern. *Electroencephalogr. Clin. Neurophysiol.*, **47**, 163–171.

WILKINS, A. J., BINNIE, C. D. and DARBY, C. E. (1980) Visually-induced seizures. *Prog. Neurobiol.*, **15**, 85–117.

WILKINS, A. J., NIMMO-SMITH, I., TAIT, A., MCMANUS, I. C., DELLA SCALA, S., TILLEY, A., ARNOLD, K., BARRIE, M. A. and SCOTT, S. G. C. (1984) A neurological basis for visual discomfort. *Brain*, **107**, 989–1017.

DISCUSSION

Dr M. R. Trimble (London), Chairman: Why are some patients compelled to induce their own epilepsy with photosensitive stimuli?

Wilkins: They find it very difficult to tell you. One little boy said it was as if God was speaking to him from the TV set. One woman described it as a compulsive attraction. They can't fully articulate the reason, though one patient was very instructive. He said that when he came into a room with the television on, if it was a good distance away he found it aversive, but if he had to approach the set for any reason then it became attractive and he felt compelled to draw still nearer. This sounds to me rather like ictal activity.

Dr J. Corbett (East Grinstead): Francis Forster some years ago in America described how to desensitize people to flicker rates. He used to give them stroboscopes that they took home and they were instructed to slow down the rate of the stroboscope gradually and this was thought to train them to tolerate certain patterns. The VDU might be an ideal instrument for doing that, because one can manipulate all sorts of patterns and rates on a video screen. Has anyone actually designed a programme for treating patients in this way?

Wilkins: No, not to my knowledge. There's much doubt about whether this treatment would work or not; it may just damage the visual cortex. However, it is true that we adapt very readily to flicker. You might like to try the following experiment at home: turn your television on its side or upside-down and you'll find that the flicker becomes very much more apparent. Obviously we are well adapted to the direction of scan from top to bottom, but whether this adaptation can be used in the treatment of epilepsy is open to question. Personally I do not advocate any conditioning trials of this kind.

Epilepsy in Young People
Edited by E. Ross, D. Chadwick and R. Crawford

Questions and answers about photosensitive epilepsy: a patient's guide

ARNOLD J. WILKINS* and JANET LINDSAY†
**MRC Applied Psychology Unit, Cambridge, and*
†Park Hospital for Children, Oxford

1. WHAT IS PHOTOSENSITIVE EPILEPSY?

Photosensitive epilepsy is a type of epilepsy in which seizures can be brought on by flickering light. Television, discos, and sunlight interrupted by roadside trees have all been known to cause attacks. Occasionally attacks can also be brought on by patterns of stripes on grills, gratings, clothes and furnishing fabrics.

2. HOW MANY TYPES OF SEIZURE ARE THERE?

Seizures vary very considerably from person to person, and some people have more than one type of attack. In some attacks consciousness is lost and there are jerking movements of the limbs. Other attacks are simply a fleeting loss of awareness and can pass unnoticed, both by patients and the people around them. Sometimes just one side of the body is affected.

3. HOW ARE LIGHT-SENSITIVE SEIZURES INDUCED?

Nerve cells in the part of the brain at the back of the head called the visual cortex enable us to see. Flickering lights and patterns are thought to cause a great many of these cells to respond. The activity of the cells is normally held in check by a biochemical balance. When this balance is upset the activity spreads through the brain causing a seizure.

4. WHY DOES TELEVISION INDUCE SEIZURES?

A television flickers because the picture is redrawn 50 times every second. Although the flicker is too rapid to see, the nerve cells respond to it and bring on seizures in some people. The picture is made up of stripes (on a colour television the stripes are really rows of dots). Only half the stripes are drawn each time the picture is created and so they flicker relatively slowly, only 25 times a second. These slowly flickering stripes are particularly likely to bring on attacks. At normal viewing distances the stripes are too fine to be seen, but you can see them clearly when you are close to a television with a large screen, and this is when photosensitive patients are most likely to have an attack.

5. WHAT IS THE SAFEST WAY TO WATCH TELEVISION?

(a) Televisions with a small screen (less than about 12 inches) are safer than those with screens of a more conventional size. This is because the slowly flickering lines are too small to be seen clearly even when you are close to the screen. If it is not possible to watch a television that has a small screen then it is essential that the television is viewed from a distance that is at least four times the width of the screen (but the further away the better!). It may therefore be useful to arrange for the television to have a long mains lead so that it can be plugged into a socket near the viewer's chair. It is not then necessary to get near to the set in order to turn it off.

(b) If it is necessary to get close to the set for some other reason, it is essential to cover one eye with the palm of the hand, so as to prevent any light entering that eye. The effects of flicker on the brain are very much reduced when only one eye is exposed. Covering one eye is also a useful technique for avoiding the effects of other types of flickering light (discos, flickering sunlight, etc.). It is important to cover the eye with a hand because light can pass through the closed eyelids. Simply closing the eye may make matters worse.

(c) It is important that the television provides a stable picture. If the picture rolls or zigzags it is more likely to bring on an attack.

(d) There is little difference between the effects of colour televisions and those that are black and white.

(e) Generally speaking, it is preferable to watch a relatively dim picture in a darkened room, although the effects of room illumination vary from person to person, and a few people are less sensitive in a well-lit room.

(f) Sometimes it may help a little to place a sheet of dark plastic over the screen. This dims the picture without reducing its visibility. Screens suitable for this purpose are sold for computers.

(g) It can be helpful to wear specially polarized 'television glasses'. These glasses stop the television picture being seen by one eye, but leave vision for everything else unaffected. As mentioned above, the effects of flicker are much reduced when only one eye is exposed. These glasses can be obtained by asking your doctor to write to Dr A. J. Wilkins, MRC Applied Psychology Unit, 15 Chaucer Road, Cambridge CB2 2EF.

(h) Some patients have an impulse to go close to the television, and may even put their noses on the screen. The attraction can sometimes be prevented by the 'television glasses'. It may also be helpful to place the television set in a position where it is difficult to get close to it.

6. WHAT SORT OF PATTERNS BRING ON SEIZURES?

The worst patterns are stripes. The width of the stripes most likely to bring on a seizure depends on the distance from which the pattern is seen. If the stripes are positioned about three feet from the eye the worst patterns have stripes that are about 1/8″ wide. If the pattern is positioned twice as far away then the stripes are worst when they are about 1/4″ wide. The more stripes there are, the worse the pattern, although patterns with as few as four stripes can sometimes be sufficient. Faint stripes are almost as bad as those that are strongly contrasted.

The worst pattern you are likely to come across is probably the stripes on the metal stair tread of escalators, and it is a good idea to cover one eye when getting on an escalator. Very occasionally, stripes formed by printed text can be sufficient to bring on minor attacks that interfere with reading. These can be prevented by covering the lines of text above and below those being read, using a simple mesh (e.g. the Cambridge Easy Reader, obtainable from Engineering and Design Plastics, 84 High Street, Cherry Hinton, Cambridge CB1 4HZ).

7. HOW DOES THE EEG HELP DIAGNOSIS?

EEG is short for electroencephalogram (meaning 'electric head picture'). Little silver discs rather like buttons are placed on the head, and the electrical voltage between them is measured and recorded on moving paper. (It is quite painless, and there is no risk of a shock.) The electrical rhythms of the brain can be seen as waveforms on the paper. Sometimes minor disturbances of rhythm occur between seizures and produce waveforms on the EEG. In photosensitive persons these waveforms are brought on by flickering light and indicate the possibility of light-induced seizures.

8. WILL I GET BETTER?

Your seizures will probably be controlled by drugs. This means that provided you continue to take the tablets your doctor has prescribed, the risk of attacks should be very much reduced. It appears that in general people become less sensitive to light as they get older. The recovery is gradual. If you have to take medication to control attacks you should expect to continue to do so for several years. But then it may be possible to reduce your medication, and perhaps stop it altogether.

9. WHAT SHOULD I DO IF I FORGET TO TAKE MY MEDICATION?

Your doctor will tell you what tablets to take, how many to take, and when to take them. If in any doubt, ask! It is very important to get into the habit of taking your tablets regularly so that a stable level of the drug remains in your body providing protection against seizures. If you stop taking tablets suddenly, then you increase the risk of seizures. If you forget to take a tablet, then take it as soon as you remember, and leave a slightly shorter gap than usual before the next tablet. But do not take double the dose all at once because the tablets can be harmful if you take too many. Changes in dose should be adjusted gradually and only with the advice of your doctor.

10. WHERE CAN I FIND OUT MORE?

The British Epilepsy Association has a range of information leaflets for people with epilepsy. They can be contacted by telephone: 0532 439393 or by writing to Anstey House, 40 Hanover Square, Leeds LS3 1BE. Chapter 11 in the following book, written mainly for doctors, provides an up-to-date description of techniques for avoiding attacks: *Recent Advances in Epilepsy*, Volume II, edited by T. A. Pedley and B. S. Meldrum, published in 1985 by Churchill Livingstone. The chapter is entitled 'Common forms of epilepsy: psychological mechanisms and techniques of treatment'. Doctors may also wish to refer to: Jeavons, P. M. and Harding, G. F. A., *Photosensitive Epilepsy: A Review of the Literature and a Study of 460 Patients*, published by Heinemann London, 1975, and Newmark, M. E. and Penry, J. K. *Photosensitivity and Epilepsy: A Review*, Raven Press, New York, 1979.

Epilepsy in Young People
Edited by E. Ross, D. Chadwick and R. Crawford

Closing remarks

D. W. CHADWICK

This has been an excellent meeting, mainly because it has brought together people from different specialties who don't meet as often as they should, not only paediatricians and neurologists, but also psychiatrists, psychologists, specialists in mental handicap, neurophysiologists and clinical pharmacologists.

Discussion of epilepsy in the adolescent years emphasizes the importance of classifying epileptic syndromes. We can then recognize that some childhood epileptic syndromes will disappear or change in character during adolescence and that other syndromes will present for the first time. Quite clearly we can now identify and agree upon the definition of these syndromes, according to seizure type, age at onset, EEG abnormalities and whether the epilepsy is likely to be symptomatic or idiopathic. We can also begin to establish the prognosis for each patient and plan an appropriate therapeutic regimen. Only then can we address one of the major themes of this meeting: balancing the risks against the benefits of therapy. From what has been said, young people with epilepsy present problems that we as doctors do not always answer adequately. These patients are of course in transition, that is, fighting to establish independence from their families and establish new relationships. Some of these may be sexual, with clear implications for counselling, not only about personal and social relationships but also on specific questions: contraception, genetic risks, drug treatment during pregnancy.

Adolescence is also the time when people leave school, ideally a well-controlled environment in which the person with epilepsy has a well-established place, where he or she is accepted and can interact with members of a peer group. On leaving school, the person with epilepsy enters a much more uncertain world, where employment may be difficult to find, where contacts with old friends may be lost. This may give rise to the vicious circle of social isolation and psychiatric disturbance that represents an almost intolerable burden for some young people with epilepsy. How can we best address these questions and provide continuity of medical care that is nevertheless adapted to changing circumstances?

This is a time of life when many people change their doctors as well as their lifestyle. Care of epilepsy will probably be transferred from a paediatrician to a neurologist. When should such changes be made? What is the optimal age? Some factors that determine this can be seen from my own practice in Liverpool. If the young person is male, retarded, unattractive and has severe epilepsy I'll get to see him when he's about 12. On the other hand if she is a young female, attractive and has relatively few seizures I might have to wait until she's 25. Paediatricians, by and large, tend to be cuddly characters, friendly and approachable. They also have good back-up, notably from school health services and educational psychologists. But what can we say about neurologists? They are perhaps less approachable, maybe a little cold, and almost certainly a little more rushed. They will not necessarily have a major interest in epilepsy and may be less interested in the person who has that epilepsy. They're often hard-pressed and some lack the resources needed to cope with the problems presented.

The young person with epilepsy is a potent argument for the more widespread development of epilepsy clinics, as has been recommended in the recent DHSS Working Party report on Services for People with Epilepsy. Young people with epilepsy require special services that may perhaps best be provided by a multidisciplinary team based on an epilepsy clinic, equipped to provide a range of services, not only medical, but including help from experienced social workers, disablement resettlement officers, and the epilepsy associations. In such centres many of the social, psychological, educational, and occupational—as well as the strictly medical—problems that confront many young people with epilepsy will become apparent. Identifying such problems is often the first step towards solving them.

This meeting has raised more questions than it has answered. In doing so, it has directed our attention to the future, and in this respect it has certainly been very successful. For this we are indebted in large part to Robert Crawford and Euan Ross for the hard work they put into planning the meeting, and also to CIBA-GEIGY for its organization and support.

Index